PENGUIN BOOKS

ALLEN CARR'S EASYWEIGH TO LOSE WEIGHT

The common thread running through Allen Carr's work is the removal of fear. Indeed, his genius lies in eliminating the phobias and anxieties which prevent people from being able to enjoy life to the full, as his bestselling books *Allen Carr's Easy Way to Stop Smoking*, *The Only Way to Stop Smoking Permanently*, *Allen Carr's Easyweigh to Lose Weight*, *How to Stop Your Child Smoking*, and now *The Easy Way to Enjoy Flying*, vividly demonstrate.

A successful accountant, Allen Carr's hundred-cigarettes-a-day addiction was driving him to despair until, in 1983, after countless failed attempts to quit, he finally discovered what the world had been waiting for – the Easy Way to Stop Smoking. He has now built a network of clinics that span the globe and has a phenomenal reputation for success in helping smokers to quit. His books have been published in over twenty different languages and video, audio and CD-ROM versions of his method are also available.

Tens of thousands of people have attended Allen Carr's clinics where, with a success rate of over 95%, he guarantees that you will find it easy to quit smoking or your money back. A full list of clinics appears in the back of this book. Should you require any assistance do not hesitate to contact your nearest therapist. Weight-control sessions are now offered at a selection of these clinics. A full corporate service is also available enabling companies to implement no-smoking policies simply and effectively. All correspondence and enquiries about ALLEN CARR'S BOOKS, VIDEOS, AUDIO TAPES AND CD-ROMS should be addressed to the London Clinic.

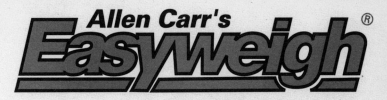

Allen Carr's Easyweigh®
to Lose Weight

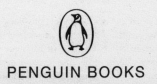

PENGUIN BOOKS

PENGUIN BOOKS

Published by the Penguin Group
Penguin Books Ltd, 80 Strand, London WC2R ORL, England
Penguin Putnam Inc., 375 Hudson Street, New York, New York 10014, USA
Penguin Books Australia Ltd, 250 Camberwell Road,
Camberwell, Victoria 3124, Australia
Penguin Books Canada Ltd, 10 Alcorn Avenue, Toronto, Ontario, Canada M4V 3B2
Penguin Books India (P) Ltd, 11, Community Centre, Panchsheel Park,
New Delhi – 110 017, India
Penguin Books (NZ) Ltd, Cnr Rosedale and Airborne Roads, Albany,
Auckland, New Zealand
Penguin Books (South Africa) (Pty) Ltd, 24 Sturdee Avenue,
Rosebank 2196, South Africa

Penguin Books Ltd, Registered Offices: 80 Strand, London WC2R ORL, England

www.penguin.com

First published in Penguin Books 1997

29

Copyright © Allen Carr, 1997

Typeset in 10/12.5pt Monotype Sabon by
Rowland Phototypesetting Ltd, Bury St Edmunds, Suffolk
Printed in England by Clays Ltd, St Ives plc

ISBN-13: 978-0-140-26358-9
ISBN-10: 0-140-26358-6

To Anne Emery, Ken Pimblett, John Kindred,
Janet Caldwell and a squirrel

CONTENTS

INTRODUCTION

While medical research continues to expand our under-standing of disease processes, it is our inability to use the knowledge we already have that still causes so much illness and premature death in our society. The dangers of smok-ing were first identified in a study linking doctors' smoking habits and their cause of death. This showed that lung cancer was almost always associated with smoking.

Encouraging people to stop smoking and lead a healthy lifestyle has long been the responsibility of the general medical practitioner, but unfortunately many doctors have not given sufficient time or thought to this aspect of their work and many have often been frustrated by the over-whelming influence of cigarette advertising, which is aimed particularly at young people.

I was first introduced to Allen Carr by one of my patients, who surprised me one day by coming to tell me that he had found an easy way to give up smoking. Since then I have recommended 'Allen Carr's EASYWAY to stop smoking' to all my patients, with impressive results. My interest in Allen Carr's method led me to investigate for myself the impact of his approach.

Having helped so many people to stop smoking, Allen Carr has now turned his skills to a method which can help people quickly and easily to lose that excess weight – something most of us suffer from to a greater or lesser degree. Having heard about and read Allen Carr's approach to this persistent problem, I was surprised to find myself almost involuntarily adopting his wisdom. The result was most welcome, and I am now able to move more easily, especially around the squash court, and I feel better for being thus healthier. I was delighted with this result, particularly as I had not been terribly concerned about those few extra pounds around my waist. Your journey through Allen Carr's book will be a revelation in discovering how simple the answer to weight control can be.

DR MICHAEL BRAY, M.B., Ch.B., M.R.C.G.P.

THE EASYWEIGH TO LOSE WEIGHT

Strictly speaking, the title should be *The Easy Way to Be the Exact Weight You Want to Be*. But that's far too much of a mouthful. If you are in the majority, your concern will be that you are overweight. However, I emphasize that my method, which hereafter I will refer to as EASY-WEIGH, is equally effective for weight gain or loss. In fact, weight control is incidental to the prime objective of EASYWEIGH, which is purely selfish: it is simply TO ENJOY LIFE!

How can you possibly enjoy life if you are permanently tired and lethargic, feeling deprived, worried and guilty about the self-inflicted misery and damage that you are causing yourself both mentally and physically by being overweight?

As you are probably already aware, I achieved fame because some years ago I discovered a method that enables any smoker to find it not only easy but enjoyable to quit. Today I'm widely accepted to be the world's leading expert on helping smokers to quit. In fact smokers who have tried and understood my method regard me and my trained therapists as the only experts.

I later discovered that, with one notable exception, the method worked equally effectively to help solve any addiction which is mainly mental, and most are, including alcoholism and other forms of drug addiction. Many who purport to be experts on drug addiction believe that the main problems are chemical addiction and the physical symptoms caused by withdrawal. Accordingly, they search for chemical solutions to the problem in the form of substitutes. In fact, the simple and easy solution to any addiction is entirely mental.

You cannot fail to be aware that today weight control is a multi-million-pound business. Every week some famous personality is promoting a video, book or piece of equipment demonstrating an exercise programme or revolutionary new diet which could miraculously solve your weight problem. There are very close physical and mental associations between smoking and eating and even closer similarities between stopping smoking and losing weight. Both smoker and dieter suffer from a sense of schizophrenia and have a permanent tug-of-war going on in their minds. For the smoker, on one side – *It's filthy and disgusting, killing me, costing me a fortune and enslaving me*. On the other side – *It's my pleasure, my crutch and my companion*. For the dieter, on one side – *I'm fat, lethargic, unhealthy, look awful and feel even worse*. On the other side – *Boy, do I enjoy eating!* You could therefore be forgiven for believing that I am merely climbing on the bandwagon and cashing in on my reputation.

I assure you that nothing could be further from the truth. On the contrary, the one notable exception that I referred to earlier is weight control. For years I had maintained that my method was not suitable for weight control – but I was wrong.

I could have cashed in on my reputation. I've received dozens of offers to endorse a variety of products, including slimming aids. I've declined every one of them, not because I'm wealthy enough not to need the substantial financial offers, but because I value my reputation and will protect it as fiercely as a lioness will defend her cubs. Quite apart from that, I haven't seen a single instance of a famous person advertising a product that didn't sound phoney. I should also make it clear that EASYWEIGH is not an endorsement of someone else's ideas. Just like THE EASY WAY TO STOP SMOKING, the method is mine and, just as I *knew* that my stop-smoking method would work even before it was tried and proved, so, by the time you have completed this book, you will *know* that EASYWEIGH will work for you.

Whereas most smokers generally put on weight when they quit, I actually lost two stone within six months. I used a combination of a regular exercise programme and the F-Plan diet. I was aware that I was using willpower and discipline. Even so, I actually enjoyed the process. It was very similar to the early stages of a willpower attempt to quit smoking. While your resolution is strong you get this masochistic holier-than-thou feeling of resisting the temptation. Whilst weight loss was the main objective in my life, everything was fine. The problem was, just like with the willpower method of quitting smoking, my resolution began to weaken, and whenever some more important event occurred, both the exercise and the diet went by the board and my weight began to increase again.

For those of you who are familiar with my method, I must clear up a common misconception. Because I am strong-willed and a positive thinker, many people suffer the illusion that my method is based on the use of willpower and positive thinking. Not so. I was fully aware that I was a very strong-willed person and a positive thinker long before I discovered my method. Indeed, one of the things that mystified me was why so many other smokers, who were clearly less strong-willed than I, were able to quit smoking using their own willpower, yet I couldn't.

I'm a positive thinker because it is common sense to be one. Being a positive thinker makes life so much more easy and enjoyable. However, being a positive thinker neither helped me to stop smoking, nor prevented me from being at least two stone overweight!

Positive thinking implies – *I know I'm acting foolishly so, by the use of willpower and discipline, I'm going to take control and stop acting stupidly*. I have no doubt that many people have stopped smoking and controlled their weight by using such tactics. Good luck to them. All I can say is that those tactics never worked for me and, if they worked for you, you wouldn't be reading this book.

No, what kept me smoking was neither lack of willpower nor negative thinking. It was confused thinking – the permanent schizophrenia that all smokers suffer throughout their lives whilst they remain smokers. Part of their brain hates being a smoker, another part believes that they cannot enjoy life or cope with life without a cigarette.

It's exactly this same love–hate relationship that people who are overweight have with food. My smoking problem ended not because of positive thinking, but because the confusion ended. I understood why smoking was just a clever, subtle confidence trick and why the feeling that it helped me to enjoy life or cope with stress was just an illusion. With that knowledge the confusion ended, and so did the schizophrenia and my desire to smoke. It didn't take willpower or positive thinking:

It was easy!

It is very difficult to convince anyone who has ever gone on a diet or a smoker who has tried to quit when using the willpower method that they can be successful without using any willpower whatsoever. You may or may not be a strong-willed person. Either way, it is absolutely essential that you understand why you will not be required to use willpower when using EASYWEIGH. This is hard to explain – an example might help.

Imagine being imprisoned in a prisoner-of-war camp. A doctor visits you and begins to lecture you. 'It's damp in here, you're in danger of catching pneumonia. What's more, you are clearly undernourished. Do you realize the anxiety you are causing your family? They are worried that you are going to kill yourself. Now you seem to be reasonably intelligent, why don't you be a good chap and come home?' We would regard such a doctor as a complete imbecile.

Yet it's exactly the same when a doctor lectures a smoker about the evils of smoking or an over-eater about the evils of being overweight. The prisoner, the smoker and the over-eater are already aware of the ill-effects caused by their predicament. In fact it would be logical to assume that, since they are personally suffering the discomfort, they are more aware of it than the person who is lecturing them.

Now it is true that with the use of willpower, discipline and dedication, prisoners might escape from the prisoner-of-war camp, smokers might succeed in quitting and over-eaters might succeed in controlling their weight. No doubt thousands have already done so. I take my hat off to them – they deserve our congratulations. However, my concern is for the prisoners who, strong-willed or otherwise, have failed to escape. What the prisoner really needs is not a lecture, but the key to his prison. Smokers and people who are overweight are in exactly the same position. The last thing that overweight people need is some patronizing lecture explaining that incorrect eating causes loss of self-respect, shortage of breath, lack of energy, dyspepsia, constipation, diarrhoea, indigestion, heartburn, ulcers, irritable bowel syndrome, high blood pressure, high cholesterol levels, and diseases of the heart, arteries, veins, stomach, intestines, kidneys, liver and bowels, to name but a few.

What smokers really need is for someone to provide the key to enable them to escape from the nicotine trap. That's what I provided. That's why my method is so successful. It enables any smoker to find it easy to quit and that's why it is called EASYWAY.

What overweight people really need is the key to finding it easy to control their weight. That is what I have now discovered, and that's why I call it EASYWEIGH!

You might well argue that it is misleading to compare smokers and overweight people with prisoners of war, because the latter are imprisoned by forces outside their control, whereas no one forces smokers to smoke or over-weight people to over-eat other than themselves. They have it within their control to correct the situation and, if they are stupid enough not to do so, they have only themselves to blame.

In fact the situation is exactly the same. The patronizing lecturers might regard us as stupid. We regard ourselves as stupid, because we know as well as they do that we cause the problem ourselves. But the fact is that if you smoke or are overweight, fully aware that you are ruining your life, and have made no attempt to do something about it, then you *are* a fool. If you have attempted to do something about it, but have failed to succeed, then you are not a fool. You might feel like one and you might feel that you are weak-willed. Does it really make any difference that you are both the prisoner and the gaoler? The only reason that you failed and remain in the prison that you have created for yourself, is that you didn't know how to escape from it.

If you were a fool you wouldn't be reading this book. You are reading it because you desperately want to escape from that prison. The truth is that smokers and overweight people do not create their own prison. As I will explain later, it is created for them by the brainwashing of Western society. EASYWEIGH will give you the key to escape from that prison, and once you have the key,

You won't need to use willpower

Did I set out to discover EASYWEIGH? No! No more than I deliberately set out to discover an easy way to stop smoking. In fact, I discovered how to stop smoking just as I had become resigned to the fact that I would never be able to quit, and I freely admit that, like all great discoveries, it was more through luck than any genius on my part that I found the solution, so I reasoned that if there were an easy solution to the weight problem, someone else would already have discovered it. I regarded myself as being in the same position as a lottery winner. To win it once in your life is incredibly lucky, to expect to win a second time would be sheer stupidity!

So how did I discover the solution to weight control? It is true that much was due to the natural mind-opening process that resulted from solving the smoking problem. For most of my life I had accepted certain facts about smoking to be true without even questioning them – that smokers smoke because they choose to, that they enjoy the taste of cigarettes, and that smoking is just a habit. It didn't really need a Sherlock Holmes to discover that such statements are nonsense. In fact, all it took was a little self-analysis. But having now got into the habit of questioning what are considered to be established facts, I find that I cannot help questioning everything, whether it relates to smoking, eating habits or anything else.

We have been brainwashed by society in general, and by doctors, health visitors, medical personnel and nutritionists in particular, to believe certain facts about our eating habits which are obviously nonsense, and which in many cases are the complete opposite to the facts.

Dr Bray, who wrote the introduction to this book, initially expressed surprise that I have no medical training. He is not alone. I soon realized that this lack of medical knowledge not only gave me a great advantage in curing smokers, but also gave me a similar advantage in finding a solution to the weight problem. A doctor is bound to concentrate on the physical harm that both smoking and incorrect eating cause, but smokers and over-eaters don't smoke or over-eat because it can kill them, any more than the prisoner remains in the prisoner-of-war camp because it's ruining his health. The only real solution is to remove the causes that make us smoke or over-eat, and that's what my method does.

The fact that I have no medical training gives me another distinct advantage. I don't need to patronize you. I don't need to use technical jargon or blind you with science. I'm like you. I've been there and suffered the same self-doubts and frustrations that you have. You won't need willpower – or positive thinking. But you'll find, as I did, that the solution is so obvious, so very easy, that you'll wonder how you could have been hoodwinked all these years.

There were three main pieces of evidence that helped me to realize that weight control is just as easy and simple as stopping smoking once you understand it.

One was the removal of the block that made me believe that the one exception to my method was weight control. Why did I believe that my method wouldn't work for weight control? Because the very quintessence of my quit-smoking method is that it is easy to abstain completely, but requires incredible willpower and discipline to cut down or control your intake of tobacco. If you applied this dictum to eating, very soon you would not only have succeeded in solving your weight problem, but would also have solved every other problem you might have had.

So what happened to clear my mental block so I could get to the truth? What caused the block? Craving for nicotine and hunger for food both lead to the same empty, insecure feeling. And smokers and eaters get the same feeling of pleasure when they satisfy their cravings.

However, the apparent similarity between smoking and eating is an illusion. In truth they are complete opposites. Smoking involves craving for a poison and will eventually kill you if you continue to do it, whereas eating involves craving for food – the sustenance on which your very life depends. Eating food is not only genuinely pleasurable, but does actually satisfy your hunger, whereas attempting to satisfy your craving for nicotine involves breathing obnoxious fumes into your lungs and each cigarette, far from satisfying the craving for nicotine, actually causes it.

Quite apart from the problem of not being able to quit

eating completely, it wasn't surprising that I thought my method wouldn't be compatible with two activities which, although they give the illusion of appearing to be similar, are in fact diametrically opposed.

However, I had made a fundamental mistake. I had been comparing smoking with eating. Eating is no problem, it is a marvellous, pleasurable pastime which we are intended to enjoy throughout our lives. What I should have been comparing smoking with was an almost equally evil and destructive pastime:

Over-eating!

I had never regarded eating and over-eating as separate entities. To me, over-eating was merely an extension of eating, probably caused by the fact that I enjoyed eating so much. Ironically, smokers believe the problems they have quitting are because they enjoy smoking so much. In fact they never do. They only believe they do because they feel miserable and deprived when they are not allowed to smoke. In the same way, over-eaters believe their problem is that they enjoy eating too much. You might well feel miserable and deprived whenever you're not allowed to eat, but that doesn't mean you enjoy over-eating.

People enjoy eating, but do not enjoy over-eating. Over-eating gives you indigestion and heartburn, makes you feel bloated, tired and lethargic in the short term, and makes you fat, miserable and unhealthy in the long term.

In fact over-eating has another great disadvantage. The guilt feelings and other problems caused by over-eating eventually ruin the pleasure of all eating.

It is important from the start that you distinguish clearly between normal eating and over-eating. Normal eating is a great pleasure. Over-eating causes discomfort both during and after the meal, and persistent over-eating leads to permanent ill health and premature death. Over-eaters are fully aware of these facts but, just as smokers are deluded into believing that they actually enjoy smoking, so over-eaters believe they get pleasure from over-eating which compensates them somewhat for the misery that follows. As I will explain later, the pleasure is illusory. Over-eaters are miserable both while they are over-eating and afterwards. That's why you are reading this book. Accept that simple fact!

This prompts certain questions: 'What is over-eating and how do you know whether you are eating or over-eating?' I fear that even by mentioning the term 'over-eating', you will form the impression that your problem is that you eat too much, and that, consequently, you'll have to cut down on your consumption. If I try to allay that fear by explaining that the real problem is not so much the quantity but the type of food that you eat, then I merely create the impression that you will no longer be allowed to eat your favourite foods.

If you follow the simple guidelines I give, you'll be able to consume as much of your favourite foods as you want to without being overweight. These guidelines will come later. Both my quit-smoking method and EASYWEIGH are like instructions to escape from a maze. It is essential to get the instructions in the right order.

Earlier I said that there were three pieces of evidence that led me to discover the secret of weight control. For the first and most important piece of evidence I'm ingratiated to

The squirrel

2

THE SQUIRREL

I know that she is merely following her natural instincts, but I find it difficult to love my cat when she is hunting some hapless bird or rodent. It's bad enough when the bird is one of those vicious starlings, but when it's a robin or a blue-tit I find it impossible.

This particular day she had trapped a grey squirrel against the wall of a neighbour's house. Knowing what agile and tough little creatures squirrels are, I didn't feel unduly concerned about the health of the squirrel. A confrontation seemed inevitable and I was curious to see whether my cat was about to get her long-overdue comeuppance. I was amazed by what happened next. The squirrel avoided the confrontation by climbing the vertical wall.

Now I'm aware that squirrels can perform fantastic aerobatics in trees, but surely they can only seemingly defy gravity by digging their claws into the timber. The wall had in fact been pebble-dashed and I assume that this gave the squirrel sufficient purchase not to fall.

I completely forgot about this incident until another time, when I watched a squirrel gorging itself on the peanuts that my wife Joyce regularly sprinkles on our patio. I remember thinking – 'Eat too many of those and there's no way you'll be able to climb the wall next time!' No sooner had the thought crossed my mind than the squirrel stopped eating the nuts and spent the rest of the afternoon burying them.

I wondered why the squirrel had stopped eating the

nuts. It couldn't possibly have had the intelligence to deduce that if it ate too many nuts it would become over-weight and not be able to escape from predators.

It also occurred to me at the time that, had you placed a bowl of peanuts or crisps in front of me, I couldn't have resisted scoffing the lot. Yet here I was, a member of the most intelligent species on the planet, wondering how the squirrel had the intelligence not to eat all the nuts.

Over the next few days I continued to ponder what had prompted the squirrel to stop eating and start storing. You and I can see the sense of it, but how did the squirrel know? Why didn't the squirrel have a weight problem? Why is it that wild animals are never overweight? Perhaps you feel that animals like seals and hippos are overweight. Compared to a greyhound they would appear to be. But their size is appropriate to their lifestyle and the variations in the climate and environment they are accustomed to. Picture a school of fish, a herd of antelope or any other group of wild animals. They might be differing sizes, but why are they always the same shape? Why are the only species on the planet that have weight problems the most intelligent species of all, and the domesticated animals whose eating habits they control?

This was the first of the important pieces of evidence: the realization that over 99.99 percent of the creatures on this planet eat as much as they want of their favourite foods, as often as they want to, without being overweight. Obviously they know some secret that we don't. Do you not think it ironic that our superior intelligence would appear to have created a problem rather than solved one, because we too must have known the secret before we acquired our superior knowledge? There can only be one possible explanation. Perhaps the fact that we are so far ahead in intelligence of any other species on the planet has caused us to become arrogant and complacent. So much so, that we actually believe we know better than the intelligence that created us. Obviously there is an important lesson that we can learn from wild animals.

I happened to mention my observation to a close friend: Ken Pimblett. He said, 'You've been reading about natural hygiene.' I confessed that I'd never heard the expression and wondered what regular bathing, cleaning my teeth and changing my underwear had to do with the things I had been talking about. Ken explained that it was a long-established theory that had nothing to do with ablutions but rather was concerned with how far Western society had strayed from natural eating habits. He went into great detail about the mechanics of our digestive and waste-disposal systems. I have to confess to a sense of foreboding as I listened to him. I formed the distinct impression that he was trying to persuade me to become a vegetarian. At the same time I couldn't fail to be impressed by the fact that a man ten years older than me looked ten years younger and was slim and trim with no excess weight.

One of the main advantages of EASYWEIGH is that it requires no technical or specialized knowledge. It relies on plain common sense. No doubt experts such as doctors and nutritionists would insist on such technical detail in order to be satisfied. As a layman, I found such detail confusing in that I found myself wondering whether the arguments were sound or otherwise and, because I did not have sufficient technical knowledge of my own, I was in no position to judge one way or the other. In other words, I found myself in exactly the same position as when listening to the claims of the latest 'magical' slimming aid, which gives elaborate technical details of why it will enable you to lose seven pounds in a week without any harmful effects whatsoever.

I found that I couldn't see the wood for trees. The technical details merely distracted me from the really powerful and important arguments: **PLAIN COMMON SENSE!** I have no intention of going into technical details and intend to rely exclusively on your common sense.

What was the true significance of the squirrel incident? Just think how nice it would be if you could eat as much of your favourite foods as you want to, as often as you want to, and be the exact weight that you want to be, without having to diet or to undergo special exercise or even having to use massive willpower or discipline. That is exactly what EASYWEIGH will enable you to do. That is

My claim!

3

MY CLAIM!

With the obvious proviso that your favourite foods are available and that you can afford to purchase them:

You can eat as much of your favourite foods as you want to, as often as you want to, and be the exact weight that you want to be, without having to diet or undergo special exercise or having to use willpower or gimmicks and without feeling miserable or deprived.

That is exactly what EASYWEIGH will enable you to do.

Surely that would be too good to be true? Life just isn't as simple as that! But before you dismiss the suggestion as too outrageous to be worthy of consideration, look at the facts: over 99.99 percent of creatures find it exactly that simple. Let's first find out how they do it.

A possible explanation is that wild animals are naturally restricted by the shortage of food supplies. That is often the case, and many will be undernourished or die of starvation. However, there is often an abundance of food but the animals do not become obese. My squirrel is an example. Another is termites. I can't think that there is ever a shortage of rotting wood. You might well argue that we wouldn't be overweight either if all we had to eat was rotting wood. True, but as I will explain later, termites don't eat wood to keep their weight down, they eat it because it happens to be their favourite food.

So what is the secret of wild animals? Let's hear about Allen Carr's magical diet. I must remove two possible misconceptions from the outset. Firstly, it is not magic. Like the stop-smoking programme, it only appears that way to some people. Secondly, EASYWEIGH is not a diet. I regret that by drawing your attention to the clear distinction between normal eating and over-eating, I may have given you the impression that your problem is merely that you eat too much, and that you will therefore be required to cut down on your intake and not be allowed to eat as much as you want to. I promise you this will not be so. In fact over-eating itself is caused by incorrect eating, which I will explain in due course.

Perhaps you live under the illusion that someone, some day, will discover a magical diet that will solve your weight problem. It is important that you first remove this illusion from your mind by understanding

Why diets cannot work

4

WHY DIETS CANNOT WORK

The evidence is overwhelming. Just think of the massive publicity we have been bombarded with in recent years propounding the effectiveness of a truly unbelievable variety of diets. Pause for a moment – if any of them actually worked, the problem would already be solved. I wouldn't be writing this book, and you wouldn't be reading it. What you need to understand now is why diets cannot work, so that if you should be tempted to experiment with the latest miracle elixir, you will know that it is phoney.

I emphasize that during this chapter I use the word diet, not in its general sense of describing the variety of food that a particular person or group of people are in the habit of consuming, but in its restrictive sense of going on a diet. That is the problem with dieting. You are being restricted! You are no longer allowed to eat either the quantity of food or the type of food that you want to eat.

When you are not on a diet, you can eat exactly what you want to, whenever you want to. Eating doesn't dominate your life but is a very enjoyable part of it. The moment you say 'I must cut down on the volume of food I eat, or the type of food that I eat,' you are making a genuine sacrifice. You will feel deprived and miserable. Food won't appear to be less precious. On the contrary, it will appear to be ten times more precious. The more precious it appears to you, the more deprived and miserable you will feel. You create an ever-escalating cause-and-effect chain reaction which is almost identical to the misery that smokers suffer when using the willpower method to quit. Sooner or later your resistance runs out and you go on a binge.

When you are on a diet you are permanently hungry. Your whole life is dominated by the thought of the next meal. You are miserable because you aren't allowed to eat and, when that precious meal finally comes, you are still miserable – either because you aren't allowed to eat enough to satisfy your hunger, or because you don't like the type of food that you are eating and, more often than not, you are also feeling guilty because you are eating more than your diet allows.

When you are not on a diet, you can miss part of a meal or even a whole meal without a great sense of loss. But if you miss a meal when on a diet, you chalk up a credit note and make sure that you make up for it at the next meal. On a diet you never consume less than your calorie allowance, but all too often consume more.

It is an established fact that the vast majority of attempts to diet have the long-term effect of the dieter gaining weight rather than losing it. If you analyse the psychology behind dieting this isn't surprising.

However, even if you possess the immense willpower and discipline necessary to stick rigidly to your diet and actually achieve that target weight that you set yourself, then what happens? Your diet is over. At last you can again eat what you want whenever you want to and, surprise, surprise, before you know it, you are back to the weight that you were before you started your diet! All those weeks, that seemed like years, of discipline, misery and deprivation are blown away in days.

Let's face it, all dieting achieves is to make food appear more precious while actually turning eating into a nightmare. It is this practice of going on a diet and the feeling of deprivation, misery and ultimate failure that goes with it that makes us dread the thought of losing weight. Accept it – **DIETS CANNOT WORK**. Our real problem is our eating habits. What we need to change is

Our eating habits

5

OUR EATING HABITS

Whether we like it or not, diets don't work. The real problem is that we've been brainwashed into adopting stupid eating habits. We are about to change those habits, not for a few days or weeks, but for the rest of our lives. Perhaps you feel that is just another way of saying 'I've got to diet for the rest of my life!' No it isn't! You are changing a situation that you don't like and you are doing it for the purely selfish reason that you will enjoy life so much more. You won't even have to wait to achieve your desired weight. You can start enjoying the process right now.

The only reason that people start off with a feeling of doom and gloom when they try to solve their weight problems is that the only solution they can see is either to go on a diet, or to start a massive exercise programme, or a combination of the two. That to weight-watchers is the equivalent to the willpower method for smokers. They search for magical solutions. At last there is a genuine magical solution which will solve your problem:

Easyweigh!

In truth it is not magic. But if you follow all of the instructions to the letter, it will appear to be so. EASYWEIGH is about changing your eating habits. No doubt you are thinking, 'Hold your horses a moment, you've moved the goal posts, you told me I could eat as much of my favourite foods as I want to, whenever I want to, and be the exact weight that I want to be. I'm already eating as much of my favourite foods as I want to and that's why I'm overweight. If I have to change my eating habits, I'll no longer be eating as much of my favourite foods as I want to!'

Most smokers genuinely believe that they enjoy the taste of cigarettes. In fact they never do. Fortunately most of them can remember that their first cigarettes tasted foul and how hard they had to work in order to cope with that foul taste. You hear smokers say, 'I enjoy the taste of a cigarette!' You reply, 'Do you eat them? Where does taste come into it?' It obviously doesn't. The point that I am making is this – if millions of smokers can be brainwashed into believing that they enjoy the taste of something that is in fact foul and disgusting and which they never actually eat, how much easier is it for similar commercially vested interests to persuade us that certain foods taste marvellous when in fact they taste bland or even foul.

A classic example is oysters – widely accepted as an expensive delicacy. Have you tried eating them? In fact oysters are rather difficult to eat. You have to swallow them whole. If you have tried them, you will be aware that you could *enjoy* exactly the same experience for a fraction of the cost by swallowing soft jelly seasoned with salt. It is true that the vast majority of those who pluck up enough courage to swallow an experimental oyster do not bother to repeat the experience.

I've picked a rather obvious example that most of us can appreciate. But the fact that the vast majority of us can see through the façade of foods like oysters and caviar doesn't prevent them from still being widely accepted as expensive delicacies. The brainwashing is very powerful and is just as effective for certain foods that most of us regard as staple essentials.

Don't ruin your chances prematurely by believing that the foods that you at present consider to be your favourites taste the best. The beautiful truth is that the foods that actually taste the best also happen to be the foods that are most beneficial to you and will keep you permanently at the weight that you want to be.

I don't expect you to take my word for that. However, what I do expect you to do is to keep an open mind. You don't have to let taste dominate your life. Taste is there for your pleasure, not your ruin. It's there to be exploited. Before you commit yourself to deciding what your favourite foods are, you need to understand more about those foods and how your digestive processes handle them.

No doubt you have already decided the weight that you wish to be. Shortly I will explain why it is completely illogical to have a preconceived notion of your ideal weight. It would be even more disastrous to have preconceived ideas about your favourite foods. You might feel it arrogant on my part to suggest that I know more about your favourite foods than you do, but at this stage I would ask you to be both tolerant and patient with me. All will be revealed in due course.

Isn't it true that the vast majority of the meals we eat in our lives are not so much a matter of personal choice, as the result of a process of conditioning from birth? Did you decide whether you wanted the breast or the bottle and how often you wanted it? When you were weaned, was it you or your mother who decided what you ate and how often?

At school, were you able to eat exactly what you wanted whenever you wanted? In the firm's canteen, could you walk in whenever you wanted to and order exactly what you wanted? When you eat at home, doesn't whoever prepares the meal make most of the decisions about what and when you eat? And even if you happen to be the person who occupies that unenviable role, in your attempts to satisfy the varying preferences of the rest of the household on a budget that makes the task virtually impossible anyway, you probably get the least choice of all.

Now you might argue – 'My partner is a marvellous cook and performs miracles on a tight budget.' So is mine, and I'll match her against yours any day of the week, but I was still two stones overweight before I commenced EASYWEIGH. I'm not blaming Joyce for that. On the contrary, her cooking is so good I couldn't stop eating.

All I'm asking you to do at this stage is to accept that most of the meals you eat are not the result of choice but of conditioning. Even when you eat in a restaurant, your choice is limited to the menu and perhaps, like me, you find that in many restaurants your problem isn't so much trying to decide from a variety of succulent dishes, but more trying to find just one dish that you will enjoy!

Are you also like me in that you like to eat everything on the plate? But how often do you decide the quantity that goes on your plate? In a restaurant you can't do that. Unless of course it's a buffet. I found a buffet actually exacerbated the problem. I would load up my plate with three times the amount of food that I would be comfortable eating and then attempt to eat the lot.

What about those delicious little snacks between meals – do we actually decide to eat them? Or are they not more often triggered by a TV advert, or eaten because we get a whiff of something that smells gorgeous, or because someone offers them to us, or because we feel bored or insecure, or because we feel we deserve a little reward? Any one of these reasons can cause us to have additional meals and snacks. These reasons all too often start a habit which leads to regular over-eating or even to compulsive eating.

I'm suggesting that our eating habits are not so much the result of our own choice but the result of conditioning by our parents and our culture, which in turn have been conditioned by massive publicity for vested commercial motives.

I'm also suggesting that you should now decide the type of food that you want to eat and when, how often and how much you want to eat. From now on you are going to be in control. Perhaps you find that a rather daunting prospect. If so, you have my sympathy. But don't worry, it's actually easy and enjoyable and that is what EASY-WEIGH is all about!

Perhaps you have also already decided that the claim I make is an impossibility and are tempted to consign this book to your waste-paper bin. Before you do so, reconsider the claim, it's quite some package!

You can eat as much of your favourite foods as you want to, as often as you want, and be the exact weight that you want to be, without having to diet or undergo special exercise or even having to use willpower or discipline.

Pause for a moment – isn't that worth a little effort on your part? Perhaps it does appear to be an impossibility, but if over 99.99 percent of creatures achieve just that, why shouldn't you?

In fact the package is far better than I have presented

it up until now. Can you honestly say that you enjoy every meal that you eat now? Quite apart from the tremendous benefits you will receive from feeling lighter, healthier, more energetic and more self-confident, you will if you follow the simple instructions that I give you. What's more, you'll enjoy those meals without having a guilty conscience.

EASYWEIGH has another great advantage – not only will you not have to diet, but you will not need to go through the even more frustrating procedure of calorie-counting. When I think back on how I used meticulously to weigh the day's allowance of butter and sugar, then stare dejectedly at the ridiculously meagre portions, it was little wonder that I was defeated before I started.

No doubt you are wondering what the snag is. I don't blame you for being sceptical. On the contrary, I'd feel that you were somewhat naïve if you weren't. I promise you that there is no snag. I value my reputation. I have no need to stick my neck out by making ridiculous claims and I'm going to look pretty stupid if you fail because I've lied to you. All you have to do in order to succeed with EASYWEIGH is to follow all the instructions. And that is your first instruction:

Follow all the instructions

This first instruction might give you the impression that the programme itself is rather rigid. Not so. One of the great advantages of EASYWEIGH is its flexibility.

I'm not going to ask you to rely on faith or trust, because it is important that you don't just blindly follow each instruction, but also understand the reason for it. That way you are less likely to ignore the instruction. I will explain the reason for each instruction in due course. The second instruction is:

Keep an open mind

This is the most difficult thing that I'm going to ask you to do. Perhaps you feel that your mind is already open and anticipate no difficulty in that respect. If so, beware – the probability is that it is already closed. For example, I said that it is important to understand the reason for each instruction. I omitted to give a reason for the first instruction. You could be forgiven for believing that the reason for the first instruction is so obvious that I would be patronizing you by giving it. Not so.

Some people think of my method as a list of useful hints which they can accept or reject as they think fit. It is not. EASYWEIGH is a complete programme that will enable you to achieve your object provided you follow ALL of the instructions. I have compared EASYWEIGH to escaping from a maze. Imagine you have spent your whole life trying to escape from a maze. I can give you precise instructions which will enable you to escape, and if you follow those instructions exactly, your escape will be both easy and certain. However, if you miss or misinterpret just one instruction, no matter how meticulously you might follow the others, you will remain in the maze. Exactly the same principle applies to EASYWEIGH.

It's strange how so many other people seem to have closed minds. To us they appear biased, prejudiced, even bigoted. But of course that doesn't apply to us. Don't kid yourself. I've always thought of myself as a fair, open-minded human being. It was an enormous relief to escape from the smoking prison. It was also a tremendous shock to my ego. How could I have closed my mind for so many years to facts that were so obvious? It was only slightly less of a shock to discover that my mind was equally closed about my eating habits.

In order to open your mind, it is first necessary to accept that it has been closed. One of the great achievements of mankind is our ability to communicate knowledge throughout the world almost instantaneously. But as John Wayne said, 'A gun is just a tool, no better nor worse than the man who totes it!' Like most of our achievements, sophisticated communications are exactly the same – no better and no worse than the information that is being communicated. Those of you who are familiar with my stop-smoking method will already be aware of the powerful effect modern communications have had in brainwashing smokers.

It's happened in practically every aspect of our lives. Let us examine some obvious examples of this brainwashing. Our general concept of a hamster is of a cuddly, furry little creature about the size of a rat. In fact the only really noticeable difference between a hamster and a rat is the length of the tail. Most people will quite happily cuddle a hamster, but the mere sight of a mouse in a crowded room, let alone a rat, is guaranteed to create panic. The impression created by Hollywood films is of the women screaming and jumping on to the nearest table, while their escorts stand unperturbed and mildly amused at the antics of the ladies. In reality, men's natural instinct is to join the ladies. The problem is, we've been brainwashed to believe that it is unmanly to have a fear of dragons, let alone rats, so we pretend that rats don't bother us in the slightest. Big Brother knows better.

But, whether we are male or female, why do we have

this different concept of two very similar creatures? Is it based on fact? How many people do you know who have actually been bitten or even attacked by a rat? No, it's because we've been brainwashed from birth to associate rats with evil and disease. The bubonic plague, the Pied Piper of Hamelin, George Orwell's *Nineteen Eighty-Four*. True, the fact is that the bubonic plague was carried by the black rat, which became almost extinct due to the introduction of the brown rat. It is also a fact that people who keep rats as pets, and even people who use rats for experimental research, find them to be clean, pleasant and highly intelligent animals.

Isn't our conception of most animals formed by brainwashing? Why do we see snakes as such evil and repulsive creatures? Have you ever seen one in the wild, let alone touched one or been bitten by one?

Why do we see koala bears as such lovable, cuddly creatures? Do you really believe that they are not infested by fleas or capable of taking a bite out of your finger, like any other wild creature?

Now let us look at some of this brainwashing in relation to food. Prawns and langoustines are regarded as expensive delicacies, particularly by me. However, in appearance they don't look dissimilar to scorpions. Now I've never been tempted to eat a scorpion – not that I've ever had the opportunity. However, even if I had the opportunity, I don't think I'd be able to eat a scorpion without vomiting. Ah, that's because they are poisonous, say you. But there are poisonous parts to most of the creatures that we eat – we merely don't eat the poisonous parts. Perhaps scorpion tastes horrible? Perhaps it does. Perhaps it tastes gorgeous. I don't think the taste would matter, I'd still throw up!

Do you think that you could eat a fat, juicy, live worm without vomiting? Yet many creatures, including millions of human beings, regard a live worm as a delicacy. Why are we horrified when we find a maggot in an apple? After all, at that stage it must be 98 percent apple! The thought of eating horse meat or dog meat repulses certain people, but do you really believe that you could tell the difference between curried beef and curried horse or dog if you were blindfolded? Even if you could, why would you want to distinguish between them unless you had been brain-washed?

I clearly remember my first-ever Chinese meal. I really believed that I was being incredibly adventurous. The mere sound of dishes like shark's fin soup or birds' nest soup were difficult to digest mentally, let alone physically. I had visions of the entire contents of a thrush's nest, including insects and droppings, being dropped in a saucepan of water and brought to the boil for about ten minutes. It never even occurred to me that the Chinese had survived as a civiliz-ation about five times as long as my ancestry, and that if the food was poison they wouldn't have done so.

Nor did it occur to me that what I was eating bore no relation whatsoever to what the majority of the millions of Chinese eat, that I was being served up a Western version of Chinese cooking. I went through a similar experience with curry some years later.

Incidentally, did you know that the main constituent of birds' nest soup is the spittle of swifts? I don't know about you, but the sight of someone spitting on the pavement, or a footballer spitting on the pitch, makes me feel naus-eous. Does birds' nest soup really taste so gorgeous that swifts can be in danger of becoming extinct because of the demand for their spittle?

If you had told me at the age of ten that I could eat snails and frogs' legs, not only without throwing up, but actually in the belief that I was enjoying the taste, I would not have believed you. I've no doubt that the fact that I was enjoying a romantic trip floating down the Seine on the Bateau Mouche with at least one bottle of wine inside me helped with the brainwashing. I'm in no doubt that I was enjoying the occasion. But was I really enjoying the taste of the snails or the frogs' legs? I'm not able to give an honest answer to that question. They were both coated with a garlic sauce.

I used to hate garlic. Now I've acquired a taste for garlic. Why is it that I can only enjoy the taste of certain foods provided they are saturated with garlic? How can we be stupid enough to believe that we can even taste a food that has been seasoned with something as powerful as garlic, when all you can taste, and all the people around you can smell,

is garlic!

So it appears that we can be persuaded into believing that anything tastes good and vice versa. Take the swift's spittle. Have the Chinese been brainwashed into believing that something that I find disgusting is gorgeous, or have I been brainwashed into believing that a genuinely gorgeous food tastes disgusting?

It takes courage, intelligence and imagination to reverse a lifetime's brainwashing. Even so, that doesn't mean you have to be miserable. In fact your third instruction is:

Start off with a feeling of excitement and elation

Perhaps you find that difficult to do. Perhaps you still have feelings ranging from slight apprehension, through doom and gloom, to out-and-out panic and utter dejection. If so, they are undoubtedly caused by the memory of the misery and feeling of deprivation that you suffered during your previous attempts to diet, combined with the loss of self-esteem caused by these failures and the belief that you just haven't got what it takes to succeed.

Get it clearly into your mind that your failures were not due to any deficiencies in your character. Supposing I ask you to stand up and raise your left leg clear of the ground. Simple, any fool can do that. Now I ask you to raise your right leg without returning your left leg to the ground so that you remain suspended in mid-air. You wouldn't even attempt to do it because you know such a feat is impossible. You might have difficulty in explaining in scientific terms why it's impossible, but you have no need to do that – you *know* it's impossible. But would you feel a failure because you failed to do it? Of course you wouldn't.

You were trying to achieve the impossible when you attempted to control your weight by going on a diet, for the reason that I have already explained: diets cannot work! Your failure wasn't due to your deficiencies, but was because you were attempting the impossible. Now it's easy to see why raising both legs at the same time is impossible, but why isn't it as easy to see why dieting is impossible? There are several reasons.

One is that the people marketing the diet confuse the issue by giving very convincing, scientific but nevertheless specious reasons why it will work. Another is that you have yourself probably achieved temporary success on at least one previous occasion. Therefore you know that it is possible. But you didn't succeed! Any progress you made was just short term and that's the basic flaw with diets. But the most convincing reason is: although we believe that we haven't got what it takes to succeed on a diet, we know many people who have had the willpower to succeed.

Smokers believe it is lack of willpower that prevents them from quitting. I say to them, 'If you ran out of cigarettes late at night, how far would you walk to get a packet of cigarettes?' A smoker would attempt to swim the Channel to get a packet of cigarettes. Ironically, it's only their strong will that keeps them smoking. The smokers that do quit by using their own willpower do so because the fear of dying from lung cancer outweighs their illusory need for a cigarette. It takes a strong-willed person to block their mind from the health risks, the financial cost, the filth and the social stigma in order to continue to smoke. After all, nobody forces a smoker to smoke. It's not lack of willpower that prevents smokers from quitting, but a conflict of wills.

It's exactly the same with diets. Dieting is a form of schizophrenia. Part of your brain is saying, *I'm fat and ugly and unhealthy*, while at the same time the other half is saying, *I really would love to eat that creamy Danish pastry*. It's a conflict of will – a permanent tug-of-war.

Analyse those people who are successful in dieting, or, more accurately, those whom you believe to be successful. Do they not tend to fall into certain categories: actors, jockeys, ballerinas, boxers, athletes etc? People to whom weight control is not only desirable, but absolutely essential. Do you not think that, because you probably give in to the temptation of that Danish pastry and they daren't do so, it will appear even more precious to them than to you? Have you noticed how many of them blow up like balloons when they retire, and some even before they retire? Get it clearly into your mind, those people remain slim because their desire to remain slim overrides their temptation to eat. But they have to discipline themselves to do so. I don't regard that as success. They might achieve weight control, but they also achieve a permanent feeling of deprivation.

Anyway, let's accept that success by dieting is impossible for you, but that your past failures were due not to your deficiencies but to using the wrong method. I've explained why EASYWEIGH does not depend on strong willpower and is not just an exercise in positive thinking. Nevertheless, it is necessary that you do think positively, or, to put it another way, that you stop thinking negatively.

Mountaineers who succeed in climbing Everest experience a wonderful feeling of achievement and elation. They experience that feeling of excitement and elation right from the moment when the seed of making the attempt germinates in their minds. That feeling of excitement and elation remains with them, not only during the considerable physical and mental stresses that they endure during the climb, but also during the extensive planning and training period. That feeling of excitement and elation is only replaced by a feeling of dejection if, and when, the fear of failure rears its ugly head.

By comparing an attempt to control weight with an attempt to surmount Everest, I might be reinforcing your belief that you are about to attempt a feat which, if not impossible, is nevertheless very difficult. Not so. Everest is exceedingly difficult to climb. That is a fact. Even with careful planning, preparation and the correct frame of mind, events beyond the control of the mountaineers, such as bad weather, can destroy their chances of success. It is also a fact that it is ridiculously easy to control your weight. Over 99.99 percent of the creatures on this planet do so throughout their lives without even thinking about it. But if you start off with a feeling of apprehension or of doom and gloom, you'll be destroying your chances of success before you even start.

Get it clearly into your mind, there's nothing bad happening. On the contrary, you are about to remove an ever-increasing dark shadow that has been destroying the quality of your life for years. The worst possible thing that can happen to you is that you don't succeed. In which case you'll be no worse off than when you started. You are in the wonderful position of having absolutely nothing to lose. On the other hand you have so much to gain.

A woman who successfully used my method said that she was so elated that she bored her friends with the details. They accused her of being a 'born again' evangelist. I don't like to think of myself as an evangelist, but 'born again', that's a marvellous expression, it encapsulates completely that wonderful feeling of being released from a world of darkness, fear, ignorance and self-despising into a world of sunshine, health and self-respect. That's exactly how I felt when I realized I had the key to escape from that fat man who had imprisoned me for so many years.

Now let's stop even considering the possibility of failure. You aren't reading this book in order to fail, and EASYWEIGH cannot fail to work for you, provided you follow ALL of the instructions, including the third instruction:

Start off with a feeling of excitement and elation

In order to help you achieve the claim, I shall be using two basic comparisons. The first I have already mentioned – wild animals. They already have the secret. But the second comparison will enable you to share their secret. The second comparison is with a car. No doubt you are wondering what a car has to do with your weight problem other than that if you walked more and drove less it might help to solve the problem.

In fact, our cars and our bodies have much in common. Both are vehicles designed to carry us around. They have very similar requirements in order to operate successfully. Neither can function without regular supplies of fuel and air. Both require regular maintenance in order to function efficiently and not to break down.

However, there are two very important differences between cars and our bodies, and it is essential that we are aware of them. Perhaps you are now concerned that you need an engineering degree in car mechanics together with a doctor's knowledge of the functioning of the human body in order to follow the text. I assure you that this is not so. As someone who still has to consult his grandson in order to record a television programme successfully, I have already indicated that I find technical jargon confusing, boring and distracting. I promise you that, even if you have never owned or driven a car in your life, you will have no difficulty in following and understanding my arguments.

The first important difference between a car and our

bodies is one of degree. The human body is the most sophisticated machine on the planet – a million times more sophisticated than the most complicated spacecraft built by mankind. Compared to your body, your car is about as sophisticated as an abacus is compared to the most modern computer. Even if you stick rigidly to the manufacturer's guide, the average car is lucky to survive fifteen years, whereas your heart pumps away non-stop for three-score years and ten without missing a beat and it will do that in spite of the fact that it is regularly abused.

Because the human body is so incredibly complex and because we cannot comprehend its intricate functioning, we tend to take it for granted. However, it is essential that we fully appreciate the true complexity of

The incredible machine

6

THE INCREDIBLE MACHINE

If I asked you to hold up your left hand, you might pause for a second before deciding which hand was your left, but few would describe that as a particularly complicated feat. In fact you could train most dogs to do it. However, imagine your task was to get every one of the millions of people who inhabit the earth to hold up their left hands simultaneously. Even with modern communications your chances of success would be infinitesimal. Yet a similar feat of coordination occurs every time you perform the simplest of tasks like unbconsciously scratching your nose.

Your body is composed of trillions of cells, each cell a separate entity, yet all working in complete cohesion throughout your life. Do you think you could peel apples, read your newspaper, play cards and answer the telephone? Of course you could – none of those tasks are particularly complicated. But would you complete one of those tasks efficiently if you attempted to do them all at the same time?

We are fully aware of the incredible skills that certain human beings acquire in activities such as sports, music, sculpture, painting etc., but those trillions of cells that make up our bodies undertake not just one simple task, but dozens of incredibly complicated tasks at one and the same time throughout our lives.

Whether you are awake or asleep, your lungs continue to breathe in oxygen, your heart continues to pump that oxygen and other chemicals through the circulatory system to the parts of the body that require them. Your internal thermostat continues to keep your body temperature at the required level. Your body continues to digest food, assimilate the necessary fuel and nutrients and process the waste products. Your immune system undergoes a constant battle to overcome injury and infection.

The problem is, because these functions are automatic and require no conscious effort on our part, we tend to take them for granted. Although it is not necessary for you to understand the technical details, it is important that you are consciously aware of the incredible sophistication of the human body.

It is even more essential that you understand the second important distinction between a car and your body:

Mankind created the car – but he didn't create himself!

You might be wondering what this has to do with controlling your weight. It is the very essence of EASYWEIGH. I have emphasized the importance of keeping an open mind. EASYWEIGH is the key to solving your weight problem, understanding the importance of the next three chapters is the key to understanding EASYWEIGH.

Mankind created the car, and as such can safely be regarded as the leading authority on what fuel or maintenance materials each individual model requires. Now this doesn't mean that you and I have to be experts on cars any more than we need be expert electricians in order to turn on a light switch. The true experts provide us with a manufacturer's guide. All we have to do is to follow the instructions.

But mankind did not create himself. Neither did he create a single living creature on this planet. If mankind did not create himself, then God or some other intelligence did. For convenience, I'll refer to that intelligence as the Creator or Mother Nature. Personally, I find it difficult to believe that the Creator is an old man with a long, white beard, who is permanently observing and judging me. I also find it difficult to believe that he wants me to worship him. The fact that I refer to him in the masculine gender might imply that I believe him to be of human form and male. To me that would be about as logical as a computer that was sophisticated enough to contemplate its creator assuming that mankind was shaped like a computer, and that just one genderless human being created all computers and everything else in the universe. I refer to the Creator in the male gender because I don't know how else to refer to him. But what is blatantly obvious is that the Creator must be a million times more intelligent than mankind.

Where do we get our information from about what to eat and when? Like all mammals, once we leave the womb we are initially dependent on either our mother's breast or mankind's bottle substitutes. Once we are weaned, it is mankind that decides what we eat, in particular our parents. How do our parents know what food is best for us? Where do they get their knowledge from? They get it from a variety of sources – from their own parents, from doctors and nutritionists, but mainly from massive advertising and brainwashing by huge conglomerates with vested commercial objectives.

Wouldn't it be nice if the Creator had provided us with a manufacturer's guide so that we knew exactly what to eat and when, and had no need to evaluate the mass of contradictory information we receive from human *experts*? I have very good news for you:

That's exactly what he did

You might find that difficult to accept, but do you really believe that it is possible for an intelligence capable of creating an object as incredibly sophisticated as the human body, to say nothing of the countless other miracles of Mother Nature, to be stupid enough to have overlooked the simple matter of a guide to advise us what to eat, how much to eat and when to eat it?

How do you think wild animals have survived over millions of years? Come to that, how do you think our ancestors survived without the benefit of supermarkets or microwaves, let alone without doctors or nutritionists? It's only in the last hundred years that we realized such things as calories and vitamins even existed.

The Creator has provided all living creatures, including us, with a manufacturer's guide. Wild animals follow it! That's why they don't suffer the problems of being over-weight.

Perhaps you suffer from the same delusion that I did for most of my life. In my early years I seriously doubted the existence of a Creator. I believe my problem was typical of the problem suffered by millions of others in Western society. I started life with an open mind. I was told that there were fairies and Father Christmas and God – an old man with a long, white beard who created us, protects us, knows our every thought and action and who eventually judges us.

It didn't take long to find out that fairies and Father Christmas were myths. I was already beginning to have serious doubts about the existence of God. After all, I had learned that you couldn't believe what you read in the newspapers about events which happened the previous day. How could I possibly believe what was written about events which happened two thousand years ago? Especially when the book was translated from ancient languages.

There was so much confusion and so many contradictions. Someone is miraculously saved from drowning – thank the Lord. 'Why does he allow earthquakes?' 'Who are we to judge the ways of the Almighty? We must have faith.' I couldn't accept this. I thought – if God gets the credit for all the good things that happen, it's only fair that he takes the blame for the disasters.

If God created all things, he must also have created hell. Why should such a kind and all-forgiving God do such a thing? If he created us, why didn't he create us all to be non-sinners? If a bad workman blames his tools, what sort of workman is it that blames neither himself nor his tools but the object he has created? How could anyone expect a child to believe or even comprehend that he would have to spend eternity in damnation all because God had botched his creation?

My young mind couldn't accept these things. What confused me most were the categoric statements that preachers made about what God thought and what he wanted us to do, as if they were in direct contact with him. If they were in direct contact, why didn't they ask him the reason for the earthquakes?

I was crying out for information but the answers never seemed satisfactory. However, the main reason why I found it impossible to believe in God was that, even though the preachers spoke with absolute conviction, there were so many different religions and beliefs, all equally convinced that they were right. If there are thousands of different religions and beliefs about God and creation, all but one of them must be wrong. I'd been given no proof that the faith I had been taught was the correct one. On the contrary, I'd been asked to rely on faith. If all but one are proved to be wrong, and there is no proof that the remaining one is correct, it is a mathematical probability that they are all wrong.

I not only lost faith in God myself, but I reasoned that everyone else must have the same doubts and uncertainties as I had – even the preachers who sounded so authoritative and certain. After all, the contradictions and uncertainties must have been just as obvious to them as they were to me. However, the real proof to me was – if you were about to commit a sin, would you really commit that sin if you truly believed that God was watching you? Perhaps you think that you would. Do you think a thief would steal if he knew he was being watched by a policeman? Of course not. If anyone truly believed that the Lord knew their every thought and deed and that there would be a day of judgement, they wouldn't sin.

Then I learned about Darwin, *The Origin of Species* and the Big Bang theory. It all made so much sense. The doubt and confusion evaporated overnight. There was no God. From the primeval soup that resulted from the Big Bang, simple, single-celled, amoeba-like creatures miraculously appeared, and through a process of evolution and natural selection developed after three billion years into the incredible sophistication of the human body.

At the time I thought that moment to be one of brilliant enlightenment. In reality, that was when my mind closed – it remained closed for much of my life. Just as many close their minds to the multiple contradictions of religious teaching because they find it difficult to accept that there is no God, so I clung to the concepts of evolution and natural selection because I couldn't accept that there was a God.

I've introduced the subject of religion. My helpers advised me not to do so lest I alienate readers. I fully comprehend the reason for their advice. Atheists might form the impression – *Allen is going to ask me to have faith in the Creator and persuade me to lose weight because the Almighty intended me to be slim and healthy*. Let me make it quite clear. I am not going to ask you to rely on faith but on indisputable fact – fact that is equally obvious whether you believe in a Creator or not. Perhaps those of you who have faith in the Almighty are concerned that I am about to question your beliefs or that I have already done so. Nothing could be further from the truth.

Was the universe created by an intelligence that we refer to as God, or was it the result of sheer coincidence? Some people see evolution and natural selection as alternatives to the theory of creation, just as I once did. How could I have been so stupid? For so many years I prided myself on having the logical, analytical brain of a chartered accountant. The truth is that my brain was equivalent to a giant clam. I had rejected belief in a Creator because I found I couldn't rely on faith – I needed proof. How could I possibly have been so blind when all my life I have been surrounded by proof.

Imagine you were the first person on the moon. There, lying amongst all the dust and natural rocks, lies a glittering diamond ring. Would you think, *What a coincidence that a diamond ring should have formed out of this chaos?* Or would you be thinking, *How on earth did a diamond ring get up here?* Now a diamond ring is not a particularly sophisticated object. It is not beyond the bounds of imagination to believe that a diamond ring could have formed naturally.

However, if it were a brand new Rolls Royce that stood alone in the dust, would you for one single second doubt that it was manufactured by an intelligent creator? Do you really believe that something as sophisticated and complicated as a Rolls Royce could just happen by chance? Only a complete idiot would arrive at such a conclusion.

If you would find it difficult to believe that a Rolls Royce on the moon was the product of mere coincidence rather than of intelligent creation, then how much more difficult is it to believe that a machine which is a million times more sophisticated than a Rolls Royce could be the result of sheer coincidence?

I now see no conflict. The hypothetical Rolls Royce on the moon would be attributed to a creator. The human species exists and the mathematical probabilities are trillions to one against us being the result of sheer coincidence. It is therefore reasonable to deduce that we were created.

Evolution and natural selection are also obvious facts. But they do not contradict the theory that we are the result of creation. The Rolls Royce wasn't produced overnight by the flash of a magician's wand. It took thousands of years of applied intelligence and trial and error to develop the discovery of the wheel into the modern Rolls Royce. If you think about it, the development of the human body from relatively simple, single-celled creatures is an almost identical process, and just as the wheel progressed and developed into thousands of different varieties of machine, so the process of evolution and natural selection has produced a multitude of different creatures. Evolution and natural selection are not just coincidence, they are obviously processes used by the Creator to improve on his performance.

There is also a serious flaw in the theory that evolution and natural selection could account for the incredible sophistication of the human body without dependence on an intelligent Creator. The theory relies on the belief that the human body evolved from relatively simple, single-celled creatures like amoebas. There is no doubt that, compared to the sophistication of the human body, an amoeba could be described as somewhat simple. But let's keep things in proportion. There is nothing *simple* about a single cell. In fact, with all his knowledge and advanced technology, mankind cannot create a single living cell. Just think of the incredible power that is released from splitting the atom. Not only is a single cell a billion times more complex than the most sophisticated spacecraft, but scientists maintain that there is more intelligence in just a single cell of the human body than the entire accumulated knowledge of the human race. A single cell consists of billions of individual parts. That's as far as modern micro-technology can take us. Who's to say that each of those parts doesn't consist of fifty billion parts?

A cell consists mainly of space with protons, neutrons and electrons orbiting a nucleus, rather like planets orbiting a star. Are stars merely the cells that constitute a galaxy? Are galaxies the cells that constitute the universe? Is the universe itself merely one cell of an even larger creature, and that creature itself merely a single cell of an even larger one?

At one time such thoughts would have been considered to be not just speculative but fantastic. But from the scientific facts that we possess about the structure of matter, whether the prime unit becomes smaller or larger it consists mainly of space with many smaller bodies orbiting a central body. Wouldn't it be rather naïve to believe that the proven structure of matter should change whether it becomes smaller or larger?

So what has all this to do with weight control? Just this – during those years in which I believed that there was no Creator, to whom did I turn for protection, guidance and expert advice? To the most intelligent species on the planet. Mankind became my God. To be more precise – scientific, expert, educated, trained, professional, technologically advanced mankind became my God. Because the arguments of the preachers were so categoric and yet so contradictory and obviously flawed, I rejected them. The great mistake that I had made was that I also rejected the concept of a Creator. I'd thrown out the baby with the bath water. It didn't occur to me that in no way was the theory of creation flawed, but merely the interpretation of those who claim to have inside knowledge.

The important point that I am trying to make is this – many believe that the human race is the result of mere coincidence. Many more believe that we are the product of a Creator, but have serious doubts about the form and motives of that Creator. Others have very little doubt. But even the most devout believers aren't able to ring him up and ask him what kind of foods he recommends. At the same time, mankind has advanced so far ahead of his nearest rivals and has achieved such incredible technological advances in recent years. Is it really surprising that we turn to human experts for advice? After all, what choice do we have?

Fortunately, we do have a choice. We can follow Mother Nature's guide just as wild animals do. Perhaps you feel that I am contradicting myself. How can I talk about the immense superiority of the human species over its nearest rivals and in the next breath imply that we have much to learn from wild animals? I not only imply it, I state categorically that it is so. Because we are by far the most advanced species and because so many of us believe that we have no direct line to our Creator, we have become arrogant and tend to regard mankind as God – or rather – scientific, expert, educated, trained, professional, technologically advanced mankind.

Perhaps we have become arrogant, but what is wrong with using our intelligence to improve on Mother Nature in order to maintain our superiority over other species? That is just the point. I believe that we are no longer doing that. On the contrary, in so many ways, including our eating habits, we are acting in direct contradiction to Mother Nature. We need to question the advice of our so-called experts.

Let's examine some of the great achievements of

The most intelligent species on the planet

7

THE MOST INTELLIGENT SPECIES ON THE PLANET

We've learned to create bombs that are capable of destroying Planet Earth countless times over. What was the justification for creating those bombs? To make war impossible. So Korea, Vietnam, the Gulf, the Falklands, Yugoslavia etc. are just figments of our imagination. Ah, but we couldn't use the bomb to prevent those wars because the bomb would destroy not only ourselves, but all other life on the planet. We've created a doomsday bomb which has failed to fulfil its only function. Was it particularly intelligent to create a bomb that we dare not use? The bomb hasn't solved any problems, it has only created a huge problem. Even if we can successfully destroy the stockpile of these weapons, how can we possibly destroy the knowledge of how to make them and prevent that knowledge from spreading? If we were truly civilized and intelligent, couldn't we devise a much easier method of avoiding war than by destroying the planet? Surely a much simpler method of avoiding wars would be not to start them.

Now let's consider some of the other great advantages of civilization – pollution of the entire planet on a massive scale, destruction of our natural environment, exhaustion of the planet's mineral and chemical resources, overpopulation, destruction of fish stocks, conversion of fertile land into desert, unemployment, drugs and unsolicited violence.

How many times have you heard football hooligans being accused of acting like animals? Such is our distorted concept of civilized man compared with wild animals. Wild animals don't act like that. They only kill to survive; even then they rarely kill their own species.

Perhaps you have heard that foxes will kill every chicken in the coop. It's not the fox transgressing the laws of nature but man. He places the fox's natural prey in unnatural circumstances. Even if a fox chanced upon a group of chickens in the wild, it would be unable to catch more than one of them. It is man who presents the prey with no means of escape. Imagine yourself a fox in such circumstances. When all you want to do is grab one chicken and sneak away quietly and undetected, all hell breaks loose. Even though the fox might kill them all, he still doesn't eat them all! It's only *intelligent*, *civilized* human beings that kill and maim each other for no logical reason whatsoever!

Just consider – it's taken three billion years for us to evolve to our present state, but it is only in the last hundred years that our technology has exploded to its present level. If history ever gets the chance to look back on those years and see them in true perspective, what do you think will be the really significant factors? The invention of the internal combustion engine, computers or television? Putting man on the moon? Or do you think that the most significant factor would be that, in less than one hundred years, the human race invented a number of ways to destroy what it took three billion years to create and, even though the vast majority of us are fully aware of the dangers, so far we have failed to eliminate even one of them?

Perhaps you feel that I'm only looking at one side of the coin. Surely I cannot deny the incredible advances that the human race has made in the field of medicine? I don't deny them. In fact I believe it is because the advances are so spectacular that we are blinded to the fact that the diseases they are attempting to cure are also the results of civilization. Rather like Lennie in Steinbeck's classic *Of Mice and Men*, who was so grateful to George for saving him from drowning that he forgot that it was George who had pushed him in.

If we are so intelligent why is it that, apart from the animals we domesticate, we are the only species that dies mainly from disease or from the aggression of our own kind? Wild animals rarely die from disease, unless that disease is due to the pollution of this planet caused by human beings or the deliberate introduction of diseases like myxomatosis, specifically designed to eliminate a particular species, which incidentally it failed to do. Wild animals die either from accidents, starvation or because they are eaten by us or other creatures.

Our knowledge of the human body has improved immeasurably in the last hundred years. We can transplant organs, and achieve mind-boggling results with genetic engineering. However, the greatest experts on these subjects admit that all their increased insight into the functioning of the human body does is to make them realize how little we understand about the workings of that incredible machine. All too often it has been shown that our limited knowledge, in the long run, causes many more problems than it cures.

Why is it that my cat can drink the water from my fish pond with no ill effects, yet I get 'Spanish tummy' merely by putting ice in my drinks on holiday? Why can wild animals not only stand, but run, within hours of being born, while the human baby is immobile for months?

So much of modern medicine is based on finding a magic pill or drug to relieve a symptom. For years I suffered from constipation. This was no great surprise to me. We are brainwashed from birth to believe that disease and illness are natural functions. We must expect to have chicken pox, measles, whooping cough, colds, flu, indigestion, constipation, diarrhoea, etc. etc. It is only natural. The doctor will prescribe a medicine or pill to cure you. My doctor would prescribe an opening medicine and within a few days my constipation problem would be solved.

But do you really believe that an entity as incredibly sophisticated as the human body was designed to have constipation? Think of the complexity of those trillions of cells. Were they designed to become cancerous? Why didn't the doctor tell me that my constipation was due to the fact that I was eating the wrong foods?

Now we tend to solve any other problems that we have in life by correcting the source of the problem rather than trying to alleviate the symptoms. If your roof leaks, do you keep out a saucepan to catch the drips for the rest of your life or do you replace the missing tile? Perhaps that example is too obvious, and perhaps that is the reason for our illogical approach to medicine – the human body is so complex that even the doctors who know more about it than the rest of us are no more effective than a pet monkey would be if you allowed it to repair your computer.

If the oil warning light of your car flashes, do you solve the problem by removing the bulb? Such a solution would not only be idiotic, but disastrous. True, the engine might not seize up immediately, but that flashing light wasn't a fault. On the contrary, it was a helpful warning that something was wrong. We tend to think of pains, headaches, coughs, fever or feelings of nausea or lethargy as diseases in their own right. They are not. Like the helpful flashing oil warning light they are merely symptoms – warnings that something is wrong with your body. So much of modern medicine is based on finding a magic pill, drug or other medication to remove that symptom. But the symptom isn't a disease. On the contrary, it is a warning that something is wrong. Often, as in the case of a cough or vomiting, the symptom is not just a warning, but actually part of the cure. A cough is Mother Nature's fail-safe method of ejecting foreign matter from the lungs, just as vomiting is her method of ejecting poisons from the stomach.

In many cases the medication that doctors prescribe to remove the symptoms actually makes the problem worse. Many doctors are now discovering that drugs like valium and librium can cause as well as alleviate problems. These drugs have a similar effect to alcohol – they take the person's mind off his problems, but they don't cure them. When the effect of the drug has worn off, another dose is required. Drugs themselves are poisons and can have physical and mental side-effects. The body builds an immunity to the drug. The addict still has the original stress, and can develop additional physical and mental stress by being dependent on the drug.

Eventually the body builds such an immunity to the drug that the drug ceases even to give the illusion of relieving stress. All too often, the remedy is now either to administer larger and more frequent doses of the drug, or to upgrade the patient to an even more powerful and more lethal drug. The whole process is an ever-accelerating plunge down a bottomless pit.

Many doctors try to justify the use of such drugs by maintaining that they prevent the patient from having a nervous breakdown. Again they try to remove the symptoms. A nervous breakdown isn't a disease; on the contrary, it's a partial cure and another red warning light. It's nature's way of saying, 'I can't cope with any more stress, problems or responsibility. I've had it up to here. I need a rest. I need a break!'

How is it that elephants can live longer than human beings without the assistance of doctors, without clothes or shelter and without being able to store food? Why is it that all other creatures can survive in the same manner, as indeed the human species used to? After all, doctors are a comparatively recent development in the history of the human race, and dieticians and nutritionists have only appeared in the last few years. Even today, we regard the practices of medical practitioners only a hundred years ago as somewhat barbarous. In fact, the human body is the most efficient survival machine on the planet. Every natural instinctive function we possess is designed to ensure that we survive, whether we like it or not, and the most powerful weapon that we possess to fight disease is our immune system.

When we remove the symptoms of a disease without removing the cause, we also remove the signals to our brains that would have triggered off that incredibly powerful immune system.

Imagine being shipwrecked. A helicopter pilot spots your SOS flares, douses them and glibly flies back to base, thinking, *Another problem solved*. You think that's far-fetched? That's just like what we are doing when we remove the symptom of a disease rather than the cause.

You might think I'm being hypocritical by knocking modern civilization. Would I prefer to live in a mud hut surrounded by a swamp? No, I wouldn't. But I'm not sure

I wouldn't trade the tax and VAT returns and the daily traffic jam in a polluted environment endured in order to sit all day in an office, for a log cabin beside a lake of unpolluted, clear blue water teeming with fish and surrounded by a natural environment abundant with wildlife.

There is no doubt that mankind has made tremendous advances in communicating knowledge and in obtaining and storing food. But what good does it do us if the knowledge being communicated and food being provided and stored is harmful to us? If our civilization is so successful, why, when the natural instinct of all creatures is to survive, are we the only species to make our lives so miserable that many of us commit suicide? Suicide is unknown in the animal kingdom. What about lemmings, I hear you say. There is no evidence that lemmings deliberately jump off cliffs to commit suicide, any more than that whales deliberately get stranded on beaches. We also happen to be the only species that has learned to cry. What about crocodiles? Crocodile tears are false tears.

The human body is truly an incredible machine. But however incredible it might be, it has a serious flaw. We need to understand

The flaw in the incredible machine

8

THE FLAW IN THE INCREDIBLE MACHINE

No intelligent person would dispute that the reason for mankind's vast superiority over other species in the field of technology is his superior intelligence. In addition to instinct, the human species has the ability to remember previous experiences and by a process of deduction to adapt previously gained knowledge to varying situations. It is this ability to deduce and to communicate knowledge, not only from one generation to the next, but from one race, culture or language to the next, which has put the human species way ahead of its rivals, so much so that we tend to believe that we are in control of our own destinies.

The basic difference between humans and other species is that the lives of wild animals are dominated by their instincts. We also have the advantage of having instincts. However, we have the additional advantage of having intelligence, and when our instinct and our logic are in conflict, we are able to use our superior intelligence to over-rule our instincts.

This is the flaw in the human machine. It has been our undoing and, unless we quickly learn from our mistakes, it will lead not only to the destruction of our own species, but to the destruction of all life on this planet.

Because we don't understand the reason for our instinctive actions and because our logical actions are based on intelligent deductions, whenever our instincts and our intelligence contradict each other, we find it logical to back our intelligence. Let me put this question to you. You have to forecast the result of a sporting event. You can seek the advice of one of two people. One is the most intelligent person on the planet, who has made a hundred similar forecasts and been proved right 75 percent of the time. The second is an illiterate yokel who has made millions of similar forecasts and has been right every time. Whose advice would you take?

We tend to regard instinct as a hit or miss affair. It isn't. It is the result of three billion years of experimentation – not of theories, but of actual trial and error. It enables birds to build complicated nests and spiders to spin intricate webs. Did you know that, taking into account its thickness and weight, a spider's silk thread is proportionately stronger than anything that man has created? Instinct enables all creatures to breed, feed and to know the difference between food and poison. Wild animals can produce offspring without the great hassle that we have to go through, without the assistance of doctors. The fact that they cannot read or write and have no academic qualifications affects them not the slightest.

I am aware that there are people who have such faith in the Almighty, and/or in the ability and ingenuity of the human species to come up with an answer to its problems, that they believe that, no matter what clouds loom on the horizon, the solution will come. Their only logical explanation for their beliefs is that the human race has always come up with a solution before. I've no doubt that dinosaurs were equally confident about their survival.

Even if you believe that there is no Creator and that mankind is the most intelligent force there is, it would still be highly unintelligent to contradict the accumulated experience and knowledge acquired by Mother Nature over three billion years. We should use our intelligence to improve our lives, not to make a misery of them and destroy them. The important point that I am making is not that you shouldn't use your intelligence, but that whenever your intelligence is in conflict with your instinct, it would be illogical to contradict your instinct.

The object of the previous three chapters is to remind you that, no matter how great the achievement of mankind, we are less than the lowliest of ants compared to the miracle of Mother Nature.

Personally, I find the most effective way to appreciate our comparative ineptitude is to set a project. Try to produce a product about the size of an acorn, which you could just drop on the ground, ignore completely, but which would then begin to grow year after year until it became the size of an oak tree, which would live for hundreds of years and would every year produce thousands of other acorns that would perpetuate the species for ever. The next time you observe an oak tree or similar miracle, just ponder for a moment on the incredible intelligence that allowed an acorn to grow into a tree, without any help from man, obtaining its immense size and strength purely from a combination of sunshine and extracting minerals and water from the earth, year-in, year-out, for hundreds of years. An oak tree isn't just a figment of our imagination, it is a fact.

We talk about the miracles of nature. They only appear to be miracles to us because the technology that created them is so vastly more sophisticated than our own that we cannot begin to comprehend them. Nevertheless they exist and we cannot deny them.

I was brought up to have complete faith in doctors. I've found it difficult to question their expertise, particularly when they are obviously intelligent, meticulously trained and so highly dedicated. However, Mother Nature, not mankind, is the expert on the human body. If your car developed a fault, would you let a pet monkey try to cure it? Of course you wouldn't! The biggest simpleton on earth wouldn't do that. But we are doing no better when we allow our intelligent brains to over-rule the edicts of Mother Nature.

You might have formed the impression that I am implying that all doctors and nutritionists are fools or charlatans. I assure you that nothing could be further from the truth. I know of no finer profession and am proud that it is the chosen profession of my youngest son, Richard. Ironically, the people who most appreciate the incredible sophistication of the human body are those very doctors who understand most about it. The more they learn, the more they realize how little they know. But if they act on their incomplete knowledge, without understanding the full effects of their actions, they are the equivalent of the pet monkey trying to repair your car. Doctors are human. I fully accept that they understand more than you or I do about the functioning of the human body. But compared to the intelligence that created us, they know little more than monkeys. This is the fourth instruction – if someone gives you advice which contradicts the advice of Mother Nature, no matter how eminent or qualified that person might be,

Ignore it!

From now on I'll refer to the fourth instruction as

The monkey wrench

Nowadays, most of us are aware of the disastrous effects that pollution from car exhaust fumes has on our eco-system and of the even more disastrous effects of breathing tobacco fumes into our lungs. We are equally aware of the disastrous effects that insecticides and other chemicals have had on lower creatures in the food chain. But why do most of us think that we are immune to these effects? Why do we seem oblivious to the effects of what we daily shove into our stomachs? Is it because we simplistically treat the things that we consume as either food or poison? OK, we know that certain foods are better for us than others and that some people are allergic to certain foods. Hence one man's food is another man's poison. If only it were as simple as that.

It is also worth bearing in mind that, provided they can obtain a sufficient supply of their favourite foods, wild animals don't suffer from constipation, diarrhoea, heart-burn, indigestion, ulcers, irritable bowel syndrome, high blood pressure, high cholesterol levels, and diseases of the stomach, kidneys, liver and bowels. Did you ever hear of a tiger needing false teeth, a hearing aid or spectacles, or a toupee, or a pacemaker? Do wild animals need dialysis machines for their kidneys? Do they die from strokes, heart disease, cancer or diabetes?

Isn't it obvious that these diseases are a direct result of what we eat? Now I don't pretend to be any more expert than you are about these matters. All I'm asking you to do is to accept that, just as the manufacturer of a car knows better than we do about the fuel and maintenance materials it requires, so whatever intelligence created us knows better than we do about what is best for us.

Now you might be thinking, *That's all very well – we don't need to be expert mechanics in order to ensure that we get the maximum from our cars, the experts have provided us with the manufacturer's guide and all we need to do is to follow that guide. But where can I obtain a copy of this wonderful guide that Mother Nature has provided us with?*

I promise you that Mother Nature's guide not only exists but was there all along for us to follow the whole of our lives, had we not been brainwashed by human *experts* and commercial interests. EASYWEIGH will spell out this advice to you, but I emphasize that it is not my advice. It is the advice given to us by the intelligence that created us, and is there for all to see provided you have the courage and imagination to open your mind, remove the blinkers and reverse the brainwashing.

The remainder of EASYWEIGH will be devoted to explaining and understanding Mother Nature's guide. Let's now get on with the programme. Fortunately, there are only three factors that concern us in order to achieve my claim. We'll deal with the obvious one first:

What is the exact weight you wish to be?

9

WHAT IS THE EXACT WEIGHT YOU WISH TO BE?

Perhaps you have already decided what weight you wish to be. I don't intend to go into detailed analysis of how you arrived at that weight. Whatever method you used, would you please just forget it. Perhaps you consulted one of those charts which tell you how to work out your correct weight from your height and age. If so, the last thing you are being is scientific. You have already fallen for the MONKEY WRENCH. Those charts are mere guesstimates prepared not by Mother Nature but by man.

Actually, those charts give you a marvellous excuse. I always maintained that my real problem was that I was six inches too short rather than two stone overweight. Those charts are generally regarded as being scientific, but a closer examination reveals them to be the opposite. Do they take account of such factors as individual bone sizes? In any event, who prepared those charts? What right did those people have to decide that all people of the same height should ideally be the same weight and how did they arrive at that ideal weight?

Forget about yourself for the moment. Do you know how much Linford Christie weighs? You don't even need to know his weight. He is obviously in superb physical condition. Observe your friends. Do you really need to weigh them to find out whether they are overweight?

Use your common sense. It isn't your scales that tell you whether you are overweight. Your scales merely confirm what you already know. It's your mirror which tells you whether you are overweight. Those unsightly bulges, confirmed by the fact that your clothes no longer fit and that you seem to be permanently short of breath and lethargic.

By having a preconceived ideal weight you are letting the tail wag the dog and creating needless obstacles. Wouldn't it be nice if you knew for certain the exact weight that you should be? You can! It's the weight you happen to be when, clad only in underwear, you can stare at your reflection in a full-length mirror and admire what you see. It's the weight you are when you wake up each morning completely rested, bursting with energy, looking forward to each new day with genuine *joie de vivre*. Your fifth instruction is:

Do not start off with a preconceived target weight

Just read the previous paragraph again. Isn't that really the weight that you would like to be? In all probability that weight will be similar to your preconceived target. In all likelihood it won't be far off the weight that chart might have suggested. But now you don't have to guesstimate. You have an exact guide to the weight you wish to be. That's the whole object of EASYWEIGH: to make things easy and simple.

Obviously nothing I'm suggesting is going to alter the shape of your nose or your mouth. I'm talking about the amount of fat you will have, or rather the lack of it, and how trim and shapely you will be. Even if you aren't completely happy with the features that the Creator blessed you with, you'll find that any imagined deficiencies will fade into insignificance, not only in your eyes, but in the eyes of others. There are few greater attractions than a trim, healthy-looking body.

Perhaps you feel that not having a definite target weight will create a problem. I assure you that it's the complete opposite. If you can accept this criterion for deciding your weight, already one-third of your problem is solved. If you cannot accept this criterion and insist on sticking to a preconceived target weight, or some fashion designer's image of what shape you should be, you will actually be saying that you would like to be a weight that will cause you to dislike the reflection you see in your mirror. You will also be telling me that you would like to be a weight that will cause you to feel lethargic and unhealthy. What's more, already you will have failed to follow every one of the five instructions that I have given you so far – that is, with the possible exception of the third – START OFF WITH A FEELING OF EXCITEMENT AND ELATION. Even if you have followed the third instruction, I'm afraid your elation will be short-lived. EASY-WEIGH is designed to help people with weight problems, not to waste the time of fools. (The Appendix lists the instructions for easy reference.)

If you can accept the criterion, but have reason to question your own judgement, particularly if your close friends and relatives insist that you are not overweight and you still feel that you are, let your doctor be the arbiter and rely on his or her judgement.

Perhaps you are now tempted to throw your scales away. No! They are a vital part of the programme. One of the reasons why we put on weight in the first place is that the process is so gradual. It's a bit like growing old – the reflection we see in our mirrors each day seems identical to the reflection of the previous day. It's not until we look at a photograph of ourselves taken ten years earlier that we can see the difference. Even then, when the ageing process is undeniable, we still try to sweeten the pill. Our comment isn't, 'Look how old I've become!' but, 'How young I looked in those days!' This is one of the kindnesses of Mother Nature – the ageing process is imperceptible. However, it's a two-edged sword. Becoming obese is also a relatively imperceptible and gradual process. If the extra two stone and the spare tyre around the midriff appeared overnight we would be shocked. We would see the problem clearly as the disease that it is and do something about it. But our slide into obesity is so gradual that we feel no shock – our minds are slowly conditioned to accept it.

By the time we've become fat and floppy we've also become used to the state. The problem is that when we reverse the procedure the improvement is also relatively gradual. Your weight, your energy level and your reflection in the mirror will appear no different from on the previous day.

As I will explain in greater detail later, this gradual process is a vital aspect of EASYWEIGH. I cannot over-emphasize that the essential strength of EASYWEIGH is that it is based on common sense. It will produce truly dramatic results in weight loss, fitness and appearance. But it doesn't take much common sense to deduce that any method which claims to produce such dramatic results overnight must be accompanied by 'cold turkey' withdrawal symptoms, lack of energy and a considerable use of willpower, together with a feeling of deprivation. In no way could such a method be described as easy.

Although the gradual element makes EASYWEIGH both painless and enjoyable, it has the disadvantage of making you lose sight of the considerable gains that you are achieving. This in turn can make you lose faith in the system. I cannot deny the fact that today I can enjoy feeling great after half an hour's vigorous exercise followed by a two-mile run, whereas a few years ago climbing one flight of stairs left me gasping for breath. But there's no way I can transfer myself back to my body in those days to realize how unhealthy I felt. I could have taken photographs every month to show how my appearance was improving, but this would have been somewhat tiresome.

However, it is no effort to record your weight regularly. You get a tremendous high every time you reach a new low – a new low weight, that is – and when you can look back on those records as I do and see recorded in black and white that you've lost 16 lb in six months without even trying, that's a tremendous incentive.

It's a double bonus when you start finding your clothes are uncomfortable, not because they are too tight, but because they are too loose! I have a favourite leather belt. Before I started the programme I had to use the second notch from the end. I now use the ninth notch. There were only six notches on the belt and now, whenever I need to tighten it, I have to cut a new notch. I can't tell you the pleasure I've had from cutting each of those notches. Part of the joy of the method is to know exactly how much weight you have lost since you started. Such incentives are an essential part of EASYWEIGH. They are absolute proof that the method works, and regularly recording your weight will provide constant proof that you are winning.

There is another wonderful advantage of not having a preconceived weight which is not so obvious. If you have a preconceived weight, you feel that you haven't achieved your object until you get down to that weight. The beauty with EASYWEIGH is that you aren't going on a diet, you are merely changing your eating habits. Once you have planted grass seed, you've done all you need to do. You don't have to sit around waiting for the grass to grow. It's exactly the same with EASYWEIGH. The moment you start this programme you have already solved your problem. You don't have to sit around waiting to achieve your desired weight. You can get on with enjoying your life safe in the knowledge that, by merely starting the programme, you have already solved your weight problem. Your scales, your mirror and your clothes will all be added incentives.

Now, assuming that you have the common sense to see the validity of not burdening yourself with a hypothetical preconceived target weight, you are in the happy position of only having to deal with the remaining two other factors that enter into the equation:

Intake and disposal

10

INTAKE AND DISPOSAL

INTAKE – the volume and type of food that we consume.

DISPOSAL – the rate at which we burn energy and dispose of wastes.

Throughout this book, the term 'eating' will include drinking, and 'food' will include beverages, unless the context is obviously otherwise.

If intake regularly exceeds disposal we gain weight, and vice versa. Our aim is to achieve a balance between intake and disposal so that we remain the correct weight throughout our lives.

Perhaps you believe that other factors enter into the equation, such as glandular problems, or changes in metabolism. 'I don't eat enough to sustain a sparrow but the pounds keep piling on' – we've all heard countless similar statements, we've probably made similar claims ourselves, but those horrific pictures of Belsen are sufficient testament to prove that such statements are phoney.

In reality I believe these factors to be merely red herrings designed to confuse the issue and to provide excuses for people who have failed to control their intake.

Don't misunderstand me. I'm not implying that people do not have glandular problems. Neither do I imply that we all have the same metabolic rate. I also accept that the metabolic rate of an individual can vary throughout his or her life. What I am saying is that you can't get blood out of a stone. Any gardener knows that if you feed the soil the plants will grow larger. But plants cannot grow on stainless steel. It is a fact that in situations where individuals cannot get sufficient food, such as prisoner-of-war camps or in areas of crop failure, the victims are grossly underweight and not the reverse.

If your metabolism or glandular situation is such that you need to eat less than your neighbour, then so be it. But doesn't that mean you can't eat as much as you want to? No, it doesn't. Don't jump the gun. Would it bother you that your neighbour's car consumed petrol at twice the rate that yours does? I'm not going to try to restrict you in any way. It will be entirely your choice.

I've no doubt that you noticed that EASYWEIGH claims to enable you to achieve your desired weight without the use of special exercise. Most people who claim to be experts on the subject maintain that regular exercise is essential to a successful weight-reduction programme. But exercise is really just another red herring. It is true that the more you exercise the more energy you'll burn, which will increase your disposal rate. But exercise also makes you feel hungry and thirsty, which causes a corresponding increase in your intake. Creatures like sloths, snails and tortoises neither appear to be over-active in the exercise department, nor are they overweight.

Even if factors like exercise, glands and metabolism do affect the rates of INTAKE and DISPOSAL, it is still a fact that if INTAKE exceeds DISPOSAL you will gain weight and vice versa. So, let's keep our minds clear and concentrate on the essentials.

Let's go back to the comparison with your car. I don't suppose one motorist in a thousand knows the unladen weight of his or her car. I certainly don't. The point is, we don't need to know. When your car gets low on fuel you top up the petrol and the weight of the car increases. As you burn that fuel the weight gradually comes down, but the basic unladen weight remains the same. Suppose that you felt, for whatever reason, that your car was too heavy. Do you believe that you would actually solve the problem by driving your car for no other reason than to burn up that precious fuel? Only a simpleton would regard that as a solution. That is virtually what we are doing if we exercise purely to lose weight.

You might feel that this is not a good analogy. You might argue that once you have used up all the petrol in the tank your car won't go; whereas if you continue to exercise your body, it will draw on those reserves of fat and you will start to lose weight. True, but in order to succeed, when you have completed your rigorous exercise and cut into those reserves of fat, you must now fast, or at least cut down on the amount you want to eat or drink. Otherwise you will merely replace the fat. However, the time when you will most want to eat and drink is after exercise. You will feel miserable and deprived if you are not allowed to eat. You will have to apply willpower and discipline. In effect you will be dieting. Perhaps you'll succeed for a while. No doubt you have achieved short-term successes in the past. They were short-term because:

Diets don't work!

If they did you wouldn't be reading this book. Anyway, why make life difficult when you can do it the EASY-WEIGH?

Perhaps you have formed the impression that I am against exercise. Nothing could be further from the truth.

I'm merely trying to explain why exercise does not affect your basic weight. I shall be dealing with exercise in the penultimate chapter.

Just as all cars have a basic unladen weight, so do all creatures, and just as the basic weight of vehicles will vary with the make and model, so each species and individual has an ideal or standard weight. Why can we see it so clearly with the car, and yet it becomes obscure with our bodies? Because mankind manufactured the car and understands exactly why we need to put petrol in the tank and how stupid it would be to squander that precious fuel needlessly. But our reasons for eating have become obscured. It is necessary that we remind ourselves of the answer to the question:

Why do we eat?

11

WHY DO WE EAT?

The answer is obvious: because we would starve if we didn't. That's true, and we've all probably used the expression 'I'm dying of hunger' many times in our lives. But can you ever remember sitting down to a meal with the thought, 'The only reason that I am eating this meal is because I will actually die if I don't?' There was an incident in my life when I seriously believed that I was in danger of dying from thirst, but I cannot remember a single day in my life that passed without food, and I suspect that that is true of the vast majority of people in Western society, with the obvious exception of those who deliberately fast on certain occasions.

Although avoiding starvation is the ultimate purpose in eating, isn't it true that each meal is prompted by a more immediate reason, such as 'I'm in the habit of eating three meals a day,' or 'I enjoy eating,' or 'Because I feel hungry, bored, nervous or miserable,' or 'Because I got the whiff of something that smelt good,' or, simply, 'The food was there and I couldn't resist it.'

We might eat for any one of these reasons or all of them. It's rather confusing, isn't it? And not surprising that we become overweight. Imagine you had the same confusion about topping up your car with petrol:

'I'm feeling a bit bored and nervous darling, so I'll pop down to the garage and top up the old car with petrol.'
'But you filled it up half an hour ago!'
'I know, I know, I'll only be ten minutes.'

Imagine an even more ludicrous situation:

'I make a habit of putting thirty gallons in the tank every Sunday morning. This makes pretty sure I never run out.'

'But supposing you don't use the car during the week?'

'I still put thirty gallons in. It's become a habit. It can be pretty messy sometimes. You see, the tank only holds thirty-five gallons. It's not funny to have to watch that expensive petrol overflowing on to the forecourt. Pretty damn dangerous too. It's caused no end of rows with the garage owner and other motorists, but as I say, it's a habit.'

'What happens if you have a week when you use more than thirty-five gallons?'

'Oh, I run out of petrol. That's why I got into the habit of topping up regularly every Sunday!'

Now you might consider the above two conversations to be somewhat way-out. You probably think that even a simpleton wouldn't act like that, let alone an intelligent human being, and you would be absolutely right. We wouldn't treat our cars that way, but

That's exactly how we treat our bodies!

Mother Nature's reason for making us want to eat is identical to the reasoning of the manufacturer of your car. Unless you supply fuel to your car and maintain it, it won't work. Unless you eat you will die.

I'm not expecting you to approach your meals with that attitude in the future. All I'm asking you to accept is that Mother Nature's only purpose in making us want to eat is that we survive. Fortunately, the process of eating happens to be very enjoyable, and the sole purpose of eating is to provide fuel and maintenance materials.

Do you regularly put ten gallons of petrol into your tank three times a week, whether it needs topping up or not? Of course you don't! If your lifestyle was such that your car consumed about thirty gallons a week, you might get into the habit of regularly topping up on that basis. However, if you had a week during which you didn't use the car, you wouldn't pump gallons of petrol into a full tank and watch it spill over on to the forecourt. Such a concept would be ludicrous. Yet that is virtually what we do when we eat! Aren't most of us in the habit of having a certain volume of food served up on our plates three times a day and then attempting to consume that volume regardless of the energy we propose to burn?

The point I am making is that the mileage we travel in our cars is not decided by the amount of petrol that we put into our tanks, but the other way around. We decide how far we want to travel and then provide sufficient petrol to achieve our object.

Now that seems a perfectly rational course of action, and our bodies were designed to work on exactly the same principle. That's how wild animals eat. That's why the squirrel stopped eating the nuts and started to store them. We let the tail wag the dog. We try to pour the thirty gallons into the tank, even if it is already full.

The point is: our bodies aren't designed to handle that surplus. For various reasons that we will discuss in greater detail later, our bodies are just not capable of disposing of the junk that we pour into them. Instead, we are obliged to store it in the form of unsightly bulges around our midriffs and elsewhere, and that's why we become overweight and obese.

You might think that the problem is OVER-

EATING, but, as I said earlier, the real problem is what causes us to over-eat, which is

Incorrect intake

In due course I will explain this in more detail. In the meantime, the important principle I wish to convey is that we use our cars according to our needs or desires. Those needs or desires might change from day to day or from week to week. This creates no problem. Provided we can afford the petrol we merely adjust the car's intake as necessary. We do not need to concern ourselves with the weight of the car or the disposal of the exhaust fumes. Our only concern is to ensure that we maintain the car properly and supply the necessary fuel.

Mother Nature intends our bodies to work in exactly the same way. Wild animals don't have to worry about being overweight, or about how to dispose of the food that they eat. In fact, their problem is usually the complete opposite – how to obtain sufficient food. Fortunately, that is a problem that Western society has already solved.

So we have now already solved two-thirds of our problem. We now don't have to ponder over our ideal weight. Neither do we have to worry about the rate at which we burn fuel and dispose of waste materials. We can now concentrate all of our attention on one aspect and one aspect alone:

Our intake

12

OUR INTAKE

I said that we have already solved two-thirds of our problem in that we have no need to concern ourselves with our weight or with the rate at which we burn energy or dispose of wastes. A motorist doesn't have to worry about the basic unladen weight of his car, or the rate at which it burns fuel, or how it disposes of the waste products, provided, that is, he fills his car with the correct quantity and grade of fuel and maintenance materials. In other words, provided the intake is correct the rest takes care of itself.

Exactly the same principle is true of your body. Only if the intake is correct will the rest take care of itself. Perhaps you are thinking, *All you are now telling me is what I knew in the first place – I eat too much of the wrong type of foods!* That may or may not be so. We haven't got to that stage yet, but your thinking might have been confused by what weight you should be, or whether all or part of your problem was due to insufficient exercise. All I am doing is to help clarify the situation. You also need to understand the effect that incorrect intake has on your body.

I sense panic creeping in. The only item left to tamper with is the type and quantity of food that you eat. OK, perhaps your target weight was an estimate of sorts, but you are in no doubt as to what your favourite foods are. Now you see the snag. I'm going to try to persuade you that a plate of lettuce sprinkled with grated carrots and nuts is a gourmet's delight. No, I'm not.

You are quite right. This is crunch time. This is the moment that will decide whether you succeed or fail. It's very important – crucial, in fact – that you understand the message. EASYWEIGH is simple, easy and enjoyable.

Let's go back to your car. If it had a petrol engine, would you dream of filling up with diesel? Even people who haven't the slightest knowledge of how the internal combustion engine operates wouldn't do that. Many drivers will unashamedly admit that they are clueless about cars. Nevertheless even the most clueless of drivers acquires a basic knowledge and understanding of cars. Do you know anyone stupid enough to top up the engine oil with treacle? Of course not. The manufacturer's guide tells you exactly what grade of oil your engine needs and your dipstick tells you the volume you need. There is no conflict of interests.

If you put the wrong grade of petrol in your tank your car will not operate efficiently. Your car has a highly sophisticated system which ignites a mixture of petrol vapour with air to provide power. The manufacturer's guide tells you the correct grade of petrol you need to use, and only a fool would ignore those instructions.

Mother Nature and evolution have produced an incredible variety of creatures over the years, ranging from amoebas to giraffes. Why is it that certain animals are so limited in their diet? Because over the millions of years of life on this planet, the various species have had to compete for food. Some species, or individuals within a species, are better equipped than others to obtain the choice morsels in times of plenty and the only morsels in times of scarcity.

The neck of the giraffe, the trunk of the elephant, the webbed feet of the otter are all obvious physical features that developed in order for each species to be better able to catch or obtain its food. Certain animals have incredibly specialized diets. Koala bears live almost exclusively on eucalyptus leaves and pandas on bamboo. No doubt pandas and koala bears learned to survive on their restricted diets because no other species found bamboo or eucalyptus leaves particularly attractive. Both species are now in danger of extinction because the specialized environments on which they depend are rapidly disappearing.

However, a specialized diet need not necessarily be a certain road to extinction. Termites were highly successful for millions of years before man arrived and, unless we rapidly change our ways, in all probability will survive for millions of years after our departure, unless of course we destroy the rest of the planet along with ourselves. The termites' diet consists of wood. Not very appetizing, you might think. Not for you or me, perhaps, but why else would termites eat it, if they didn't enjoy it? Having learned to digest wood, termites have guaranteed themselves an everlasting supply of free and available meals, always providing the human species will one day refrain from this terrible practice of converting the whole planet into concrete jungles or deserts.

The external developments that have occurred in the various species are often not only obvious, but spectacular. But the giraffe's legs and neck and the elephant's trunk and tusks didn't grow to their present length overnight. These changes occurred gradually over hundreds of thousands of years. As the creatures' external features evolved, so their internal organs, including their digestive systems, evolved to keep pace. We have one stomach but a cow has four.

Just as the manufacturer of your car recommends an exact specification in the form of fuel and maintenance materials, so Mother Nature has provided each creature with an exact package or variety of packages of food. You've heard the expression – one man's food is another man's poison. A more apt expression would be – one species' food is another species' poison.

The car manufacturer recommends the fuel suitable for the engine. But with evolution it appears to be the other way around – a creature's digestive system adapts to suit the supply of food available. In fact this difference is more apparent than real. The man who built the first petrol engine didn't build it first and then go out to discover oil. He developed the engine to accommodate the source of fuel and, just like evolution, both the engines and the oil-refining process have evolved considerably since that first engine.

The important point which follows on is this: engines will continue to develop but, whatever engine you happen to have in your car at the moment, you need to provide the fuel and maintenance materials designed for it. Exactly the same principle applies to your digestive system. No doubt in another hundred thousand years the human will also have evolved. But our lives will be much longer and happier if we cater for the digestive system that we have and that has hardly changed since our ancestors first left the trees.

Another related point – if we were to put diesel fuel in a petrol engine, the car wouldn't go. Yet we can eat an incredible variety of food and still survive. So how can I possibly argue that only certain food packages were designed for the human species? But isn't that why you are reading this book? You are eating the wrong food packages. That's why you are overweight, lethargic and fat.

Yes, we survive, but that is only because our bodies are incredibly ingenious, infinitely more so than any car. In fact, so ingenious is the system that if you swallow broken glass or a coin, your body is able to dispose of it; but you wouldn't make coins a part of your regular diet. This is one of the beauties of the system. Our bodies can process certain quantities of junk food without any adverse effects whatsoever. But is that any excuse to treat our bodies like waste-disposal units? **WILD ANIMALS EAT ONLY NATURAL FOODS!**

What is a natural food?

13

WHAT IS A NATURAL FOOD?

A natural food is any food that you eat in its natural state. In other words – it hasn't been tampered with by man. This means that it hasn't been cooked, refined, frozen, pickled, bottled, preserved, sweetened, flavoured, canned, smoked, mixed or whatever. And it contains no additives whatsoever, including salt and pepper.

Forgive me if this is incorrectly anticipating your thoughts: 'What! We can no longer cook food? We can no longer season it or enhance the taste by the addition of delicious sauces?' Of course you can. One of the beauties of EASYWEIGH is that there are no restrictions! All I'm asking you to do is to try to think what foods you can eat in their natural state, that you don't have to cook or process, and that not only taste marvellous, but require no seasoning or sauces to enhance the taste. Isn't it only fresh fruit, vegetables and nuts? I'm not saying that you will enjoy all varieties of such foods. What I am saying is that no other foods are enjoyable or palatable to human beings in their natural state.

Let's just consider how much tampering is involved in a simple snack like a slice of toast with butter and jam. The wheat is milled and the flour is refined. Yeast and other ingredients are added and the dough is cooked to provide the loaf. The slice of bread is then reheated. The butter is processed from cows' milk. Perhaps you regard cows' milk as a natural food. It is, but only for calves. That milk is then pasteurized, homogenized and heated, then processed again to provide the butter. The butter is refrigerated to keep it from becoming rancid. The jam is processed fruit which has been boiled with sugar, which itself has been refined and processed. Now that's an incredible amount of interference for just one little snack.

You might well be thinking – *So what? Each bit of tampering improves the quality of the food*. Does it? Or is it the MONKEY WRENCH? Has it merely reduced nutritious food to junk? We'll discuss that later. The point I'm making at this stage is that although nature has provided us with a variety of foods in their natural state, just consider the food that you have consumed over the past few days and ask yourself how much of it was natural. You'll probably find, as I did, that you rarely eat any food in its natural state.

We tend to categorize the various species into carnivores, herbivores or omnivores. Some animals, such as goats, have the constitution to eat almost anything and survive. However, the animal that has by far the greatest variety of diet is the human being, or, more accurately, Western-society man. This is because man had the intelligence to discover, reach, trap, cultivate, preserve, store, cook, season, refine and combine a greater variety of foods than all other species on the planet combined. A goat might be better equipped to digest foods like caviar but it seldom gets the opportunity.

Western man is indeed fortunate to be at the top of the survival tree and to have his pick of an incredible variety of delicious and nutritious foods. No doubt termites had to learn to eat wood because no other creatures either fancied it or had the stomach to eat it. It is this last phrase that I want you to concentrate on. Just as natural selection gradually altered the external physical characteristics of different creatures, so that they became better equipped to discover, reach or catch their food, so the far more complicated internal chemical and physical processes – of digesting food, selecting and extracting the vital nutrients from the waste, distributing the energy to where it is needed and disposing of that waste – had to alter and adapt to the changing diet.

Goats are renowned for their strong constitutions. But as far as variety of intake is concerned, the human species is in a class of its own. Other omnivores will usually eat just one variety of food at any particular meal. We not only eat a variety of courses during one meal, but each course often consists of a number of different types of food, with added sauces and flavourings. Indeed, often each mouthful contains many different types of food. Once we have swallowed that mouthful, because our digestive systems are automatic, it ceases to be our problem. Our digestive systems have always coped, so why not let them get on with it?

Supposing you ran out of petrol and I said, 'Wait a minute. A car runs on a mixture of petrol and air. You've got a plastic bucket in your boot. I happen to know that plastic, like petrol, is a by-product of crude oil. If we cut the bucket up into small pieces, shove them into the petrol tank and then blow air into the tank, we have solved the problem.' Would you think I was a genius or a candidate for the funny farm? Anyone would know that this was nonsense. Yet this is virtally what the majority of us routinely do to our bodies throughout our lives. I shall refer to this as

The plastic bucket syndrome

14

THE PLASTIC BUCKET SYNDROME

Our cars are expensive machines. We feel perturbed at the slightest sign of trouble. Yet our most precious possession, the vehicle on which we depend for the length and quality of our lives, we treat rather like a waste-disposal unit. The restricted diets of koala bears and pandas threaten them with extinction, but it doesn't necessarily follow that a wide variety of food guarantees survival. On the contrary, this incredible variety is the cause of the premature death of millions of human beings.

We naïvely categorize anything we are capable of eating as either food or poison. Providing it is food, we feel entitled to eat it without the slightest consideration for how our bodies can digest it, extract the nutrients and dispose of the wastes.

Perhaps you feel that the plastic bucket syndrome is an exaggeration. I promise you that it is not. Our digestive systems are highly complicated and sophisticated.

The process starts before we even put the food into our mouths. We first prepare our food by removing the inedible pieces or cooking it in order to make it more digestible. There are ample adages or proverbs that the human race has accumulated over the years in relation to the procedure. 'Don't bite off more than you can chew.' This might appear to be obvious, but why? We can swallow quite large lumps of food without chewing them. It's only obvious when you connect the lack of chewing with indigestion and constipation. This knowledge has led to 'Chew each mouthful one hundred times!' Have you ever tried chewing a bite of banana one hundred times?

When we chew the food it is mixed with saliva, which also plays its part. The mixture is then swallowed and passes down to our stomachs, where it is broken down further by means of digestive juices. These juices vary according to different types of food, as do the time and energy taken to digest each type of food. Whether properly digested or otherwise, food is then passed into the intestines. It is only at this stage that the vital chemicals can be extracted – providing, that is, that the food has been properly digested – and the process of distributing those chemicals and disposing of the waste products can begin.

Ironically, it is the so-called experts who create the plastic bucket syndrome. We have been taught that from birth we need protein and calcium to build strong, healthy muscles, bones and teeth. What's the best way to obtain protein? It's so obvious – eat meat. So we eat cows. But is it so obvious? Where did the cow get its protein from? Cows are vegetarians. What are the largest land animals? Elephants, giraffes, hippos, rhinos, horses, bullocks, gorillas etc. – all herbivores. If these so-called experts recommend that we eat muscles in order to obtain our protein, surely the logical consequence is to advise us to eat bones and teeth to obtain iron and calcium. Or to go one stage further, why don't we just eat iron filings and chalk? Because that would obviously be ludicrous. So the so-called experts advise us to eat cheese or to drink milk in order to obtain that vital calcium. That's equally ludicrous, but not so obvious. Which animal has the largest teeth? Wouldn't you agree that the tusks of a bull elephant are far larger than any teeth you've ever seen?

Do you realize how many pints of milk and pounds of cheese an elephant has to eat to produce and maintain those huge tusks? Absolutely none. An elephant obtains all its energy, power and immense strength from eating vegetation.

Understanding the plastic bucket syndrome is a vital part of EASYWEIGH. The next time a so-called expert advises you to eat a particular food or to take a particular pill because it contains the vitamins or nutrients that you are lacking, think of the plastic bucket in your petrol tank. Our digestive systems just don't work that way. The carburettors in our cars are highly sophisticated pieces of equipment designed to convert a mixture of petrol and air into fuel. The correct grade of petrol is the package specifically designed for it. Our digestive systems are infinitely more complicated and sophisticated than our carburettors. Mother Nature has provided specially designed food packages for all creatures on this planet, and if we ignore those packages or tamper with them before eating them, how can we possibly expect to remain energetic and healthy?

Perhaps you are concerned about vitamin deficiency, obtaining a balanced diet or calorie counting. Have no fear, these are problems created by civilized man because we don't follow Mother Nature's guide. Always remember – life has survived on this planet for millions of years without these problems. Wild animals survive today without them.

I'm aware that it is very difficult not to heed the advice of a nutritionist or doctor who has been trained to understand the functioning of the human body. But remember the fourth instruction: the MONKEY WRENCH. If an expert gives you advice which contradicts the advice of the intelligence that created us, it will also contradict your common sense. That expert might just as well be telling you to top up your tank with a plastic bucket!

Perhaps you are thinking that wild animals don't have to use their common sense and they have no idea how their digestive systems work, yet they seem able to eat a variety of foods without any harmful effects, so why can't we? That is the very point I'm trying to make. We don't need to know how our cars work. All we need to do is to follow the manufacturer's guide. Wild animals don't need to know how their digestive systems work. In a way they are fortunate – they do not have the intelligence to contradict the manufacturer's guide. They merely eat the packages that Mother Nature's guide tells them to eat. Our problem is that we have been brainwashed to believe that man, and not Mother Nature, is the expert on what we should eat. We've allowed our intelligence to interfere with and to supersede our natural instincts.

The only reason why you need to understand your digestive system now is to realize the stupidity of not following Mother Nature's guide and the consequences that will ensue if you continue to ignore it.

As a chain-smoker, the risk of contracting lung cancer did not make me quit. I took the attitude that if you were lucky enough to get away with it, that's exactly what you did – you got away with it completely. However, I'm convinced I would have quit immediately could I have seen the effect that smoking was having inside my body. I'm not talking about the staining of my lungs, but the coagulation of my blood, the progressive blocking-up of my blood vessels, the incredible strain on my poor heart as it bravely fought to pump the ever-thickening gunge around the ever-narrowing apertures of my arteries and veins without missing a single beat, let alone having a whole day off.

I'm grateful that the human body is so incredibly strong that it enabled me to survive the punishment that I inflicted upon it. However, in no way would I have subjected my body to that ordeal if I'd had the slightest idea of the pressure I was putting it under. I really couldn't have blamed it if it had turned round at any stage in my life and said, 'Look! This is supposed to be a partnership. If you couldn't give a damn about what happens to you, why should I keep banging my head against a brick wall?' If you were lucky enough to own a Rolls Royce, would you expect your repair man to take an interest if you continually poured salt water over it? What's that? You are not lucky enough to own a Rolls Royce? You own a machine that is a billion times more valuable and sophisticated than a Rolls Royce:

Your body

For most of my life I've been following exactly the same head-in-the-sand procedure with my eating habits as I used to with my smoking addiction. I was under exactly the same illusion that I was sacrificing longevity for a shorter and much more enjoyable life. How I could have believed that a life of being overweight, lethargic and short of breath, frequently suffering from indigestion and constipation, and permanently feeling guilty and deprived, was sweeter is hard to imagine. The only justification I can give is the excuse that, as with smoking, I thought I had no choice – and if you have no choice you might as well make the best of a bad job.

Fortunately, with both smoking and eating, you do have

a choice. My only regret is that in both cases it took me so long to counter the misinformation that society had so effectively indoctrinated me with.

It's incredible how fussy we are about the liquids that we pour into our cars, yet we treat our bodies like huge waste-disposal units, regularly shoving all manner of food in all manner of combinations down one end and leaving our bodies to cope with it, without giving a single thought to the immense strain we are putting them under. My attitude was: 'Well, so far so good!' – exactly the same comment that the man who fell from the roof of a skyscraper was heard to make as he passed the tenth floor.

Now that I have acquired some knowledge of the digestive processes, the mystery to me is not that I just suffered inconvenience from indigestion and constipation, but that my body actually survived the seemingly impossible task that I subjected it to daily for over fifty years. The human body is indeed an incredible machine! Why do we go out of our way to make life so difficult for it? After all, our happiness and longevity depend upon it. We need to work in harmony with our bodies, and to do that we need to facilitate their natural functions and not go out of our way to impede them. To do that, we need a basic knowledge of how the system works.

Am I patronizing you by suggesting that your body is your most valuable asset? You know that as well as I do! So why is it that we go to so much trouble and expense to protect our cars. We wouldn't pour salt water over them daily. So why do we daily poison and punish our most precious asset? Do we really do it out of sheer stupidity, or is not a more rational explanation that we do it out of ignorance and confusion? With our car, we have the manufacturer's guide and know exactly what to do, whereas our eating habits are a conglomeration of tradition, ignorance, commercialism, advertising, convenience, contradiction and confusion. We have not just one guide but thousands.

Have you ever had that marvellous feeling of operating a spanking new lawn-mower? The blade scythes cleanly and effortlessly through the grass. Occasionally the blade hits an unnoticed stone. It has the same effect on us as grating the car gears. We know that the lawn-mower isn't built to cut rocks and do all we can to make sure it doesn't try to.

Start thinking of your body as a machine designed to carry out a multitude of functions. One of the most important functions is your digestive system. We eat to provide fuel or energy to enable the machine to operate. Unlike a car, your body is self-repairing and self-maintaining, and requires a variety of chemicals to replace the millions of cells that die each day. These essential chemicals are also provided by our food.

At least once in our lives, the parents amongst us have been through the trauma of a baby or young child having swallowed a coin, a safety pin or some other equally frightening and indigestible object. Is the usual outcome death or a major operation? No, usually the object is miraculously ejected a few days later from the other end, leaving both baby and coin none the worse for wear.

I suppose it is such incidents, reinforced by experiences of idiots that eat fire, broken glass and even metal, but still survive, that lead us to believe that we can eat almost anything and survive. Our bodies are indeed miraculous. They can survive and cope with such isolated traumas, just as your lawn-mower can survive the occasional stone.

But how long do you think your lawn-mower would last if you tried to mow Pebble Beach?

The mere prospect of attempting to do such a thing is almost unthinkable. Yet that is effectively what most members of Western society do to the most precious machine that they possess – **EVERY DAY OF THEIR LIVES!**

The principles for efficient operation of the digestive system are identical to those of any other successful production line. A regular supply of the right quantity and quality of raw materials, and a smooth processing and distribution of both product and waste, without shortage of supplies, overloading, clogging-up or breakdowns at any stage of the process.

Let's find out more about how Mother Nature's guide works. Have you ever wondered:

How do wild animals distinguish between food and poison?

15

HOW DO WILD ANIMALS DISTINGUISH BETWEEN FOOD AND POISON?

I said earlier that wild animals instinctively know the difference between food and poison. Have you ever wondered how they do it? After all, it's easy for us, we are intelligent human beings. We make sure that we don't feed poisons to our children and, if we are sensible, we ensure that poisons are kept safely locked up out of their reach. We are taught what is food and what is poison. But how do wild animals know?

For a moment, put yourself in the place of Mother Nature. You've created this incredible variety of species. How do you ensure that they don't all poison themselves? They've all got specialized digestive systems designed to consume specialized food packages. How would you ensure that they eat the food packages most suited to them? One way would be to provide them with senses. You could give them sight: that looks like food. You could give them touch: it looks like food but feels like a rock. You could give them a sense of smell and taste. If it smells and tastes awful, it's poison. If it smells and tastes good, it's food. And if it smells and tastes marvellous, that's the food package designed for me.

Does such a system sound sensible to you? Of course it does, it's so obvious! So why does Sod's Law have to rear its ugly head once more? Why has our Creator made all the things that are so bad for us – like smoking, alcohol, juicy steaks, double cream and exotic sweets – appear so pleasurable? Why didn't he make the things that are bad for us taste awful and the things that are good for us taste great? I have very good news for you:

That is exactly what he did!

It's only the influence of man that has brainwashed us into believing there is some genuine pleasure in poisoning ourselves with nicotine, alcohol or junk foods. The beautiful truth is:

The foods that taste the best are the most beneficial to you

Remember, that's the sole object of taste – that's how wild animals know what to eat. What more ingenious or simple guide could there be?

Have you ever noticed how your pet cat will first sniff her food, then gingerly touch it with her nose, then demean herself by actually sampling the merest scrap before either scoffing down the rest or walking away with her nose in the air as if you were feeding her poison? She also has her tail in the air to let you know what she thinks of the food. The ingratitude of it used to infuriate me. After all, she wasn't even my cat. She was a stray that just walked into our house one day and decided it would suit her purposes until she found something better. Didn't she realize that I had bought her the finest and most expensive cat food on the market, and that the cat-food manufacturers and I were far more intelligent than she was and knew far better than she did what food was good for her?

How stupid could I have been? To believe that a cat-food manufacturer and I knew better than my cat about her favourite foods is about as logical as a man, no matter how qualified he thinks he is, advising a woman of the best position to adopt during labour.

In fact, the Creator's system is so sophisticated there is no need to stamp 'sell-by' dates on his packages. When natural foods begin to rot, they start to look awful, feel awful, smell awful and taste awful. A rotten apple is a classic example.

Now I'm not clever enough to know how the Creator managed the intricate details. In fact, so stupid am I that I spent over fifty years on this planet before the problem even dawned on me, let alone the solution. How do wild animals know the difference between food and poisons? I think if my complacent, intelligent and educated mind hadn't prevented me from asking the question, the answer would have been so simple and obvious:

Foods taste and smell good! Poisons taste and smell foul!

Taste is the main indication of the correct foods that we should eat. Smell is closely associated with taste. Any good chef knows that appearance and texture are also important. I find that when a banana becomes over-ripe, it still smells good and tastes good, but the effect is spoiled by the mushy appearance and feel. Even the fifth sense – hearing – can enter into the equation. I love the sound of bacon being fried to a crisp. I find the smell even more gorgeous. But I find the taste salty and the appearance offensive, either because it's swimming in fat or because I find the crispy look indigestible – and bacon never fails to give me indigestion.

For a food to be acceptable, it doesn't need to satisfy all the senses. But if one of your senses is anti – beware. In particular, beware of any substance which smells good, but doesn't taste good, like tobacco and coffee. This is usually the sign of an addictive drug combined with a poison. Although smell and taste are closely linked, do not assume that because you like the smell you must automatically like the taste. Try drinking your favourite perfume. On second thoughts, don't!

Just as the manufacturer's guide tells us the exact grade of petrol to put in our car tanks, so our senses tell us what type of food to eat, and assuming they are all in harmony there is no problem. Perhaps our most important sense is our sixth sense. It doesn't matter whether you call it intuition or instinct. It's used when your logical mind arrives at one conclusion but your instinct contradicts that conclusion. Remember, your instinct is the result of three billion years of logic, and remember that wild animals don't have these problems because they have no logic and have to rely on instinct. What could be more logical?

This is why you will find EASYWEIGH so acceptable. Because, for the first time in your life when contemplating weight problems, there will be no contradiction between your logical mind and your instincts. In fact, the method explains why logic and instinct are in true harmony, thus removing the schizophrenia that we suffer about weight problems. The uncertainty, the doubt and the confusion are removed because you realize that the foods that were designed to make you feel fit and healthy happen to taste the best. No longer will you suffer the dichotomy of craving the foods that you know are the most harmful to you.

At this stage I do not expect you to understand why the foods which taste the best are the ones most beneficial to you. However, just as the pleasure in tobacco is a subtle illusion, so is the belief that harmful foods taste good. However, just as we must learn to walk before we can run, first you need to understand more about how the manufacturer's guide works. In due course I will explain how the illusion was perpetrated and how to correct it. In the meantime I would ask you to accept the concept that the foods that taste and smell the best are the most beneficial to you. This is Mother Nature's guide, and this is why wild animals do not have the eating problems that we do.

Now we haven't yet identified the exact food packages most suitable for the human species, but we have established the principles involved in deciding what to eat. But

How do we know when to start and when to stop eating?

16

HOW DO WE KNOW WHEN TO START AND STOP EATING?

How do the car manufacturers solve the problem? They provide a petrol gauge, with additional sophistications like flashing warning lights in case we forget to look at the gauge, and a device on the petrol pump to switch it off when the tank is full.

How does Mother Nature solve this problem? Let us play at being the Creator for a moment. You've created this incredible variety of species. By giving them senses such as taste and smell you successfully prevent them from poisoning themselves. But how do you ensure they all eat in the first place? After all, unless each creature consumes sufficient and regular quantities of food it will die. It's easy for human beings – our parents make sure we eat and, by the time we leave them, we understand that we have to eat to survive. All we have to do is to visit the supermarket once a week, take food out of the fridge and pop it into the microwave. But for most wild creatures, obtaining food is an exceedingly arduous and dangerous pastime which can involve hours, even days, of patience, exhaustion and frustration, and which all too often ends up with them becoming a meal rather than obtaining one. So how would you ensure that all wild animals ate regularly?

The solution is simple. You provide each and every one of them with an ingenious device called **HUNGER**. That's how wild animals know when to eat: when they feel hungry! That's how they know when to stop eating: when they no longer feel hungry.

The solution may be simple, but let that not distract us from the ingenuity of the device. We tend to regard hunger as a rather unpleasant sensation, particularly if we've spent years fighting the battle of the bulge. The reality is that hunger should provide us with more hours of pleasure throughout our lives than any other single activity.

Why do I describe hunger as an ingenious device? Surely being hungry is not a particularly desirable state to be in? If you live in the Third World and are starving, I agree with you. Even then, hunger isn't the real evil – hunger is merely telling you that you must get food, otherwise you will die. It is the inability to satisfy that hunger which is the real evil. However, this book isn't designed to solve the problem of starvation. It is designed to solve the exact opposite problem.

Can you remember when you were last really hungry? Unless you belong to a faith in which fasting is a regular practice, it was probably the last time you were on a diet. How long did you go without food? A month, a week, a day? OK, perhaps you've never been in danger of starving; even so, how can I describe hunger as providing us with pleasure?

Let's study hunger more closely. What is hunger? It works rather like our petrol gauge. As we burn up energy and as our trillions of cells die and regenerate, our stocks of energy and maintenance materials need to be replaced. Just as when we have recently filled our petrol tanks we don't keep looking at the gauge to see whether we need to top up again, so when we finish a meal our stocks have been replenished and we don't feel hungry for a while.

I use myself as an example. Except that I always eat breakfast now, my eating habits are still the same as when I was a smoker. After breakfast I do not eat again until dinner, which is usually about 6 p.m. You might be thinking that I will be recommending that you, too, should limit yourself to two meals per day. Not so – remember, there are no restrictions. I eat two meals a day, not for reasons of willpower or discipline, but for the purely selfish reason that it suits my lifestyle; I would find it inconvenient to interrupt the flow of my work. Now hunger is nature's way of saying, 'You need to top up on fuel and nutrients.' Obviously, between breakfast and dinner these stocks are gradually being depleted, yet I am not aware of being hungry – I suffer no inconvenience whatsoever. On the contrary, as I have already explained, I would find it inconvenient to eat during the day. Please do not be alarmed. I'm not going to suggest that you adopt the same procedure. Let me remind you of the claim: I make no restrictions whatsoever! The point I am making is that I am not aware of being hungry during the intervening period.

However, if I have occasion to go out during the day and I get the whiff of food cooking, or if I'm working late and the smell of one of Joyce's culinary delights comes wafting up from the kitchen, then that gradual, chemical depletion, which is continuous in our bodies throughout our lives, sets off a flashing warning light to my brain – **YOU ARE HUNGRY! YOU MUST EAT!** This is why hunger is such a wonderful, ingenious device. If we follow Mother Nature's guide, there is no aggravation. Initially, we aren't even aware that we are hungry. And when we become aware, provided we are allowed to satisfy that hunger, we can enjoy the immense pleasure that satisfaction gives.

Hunger is infinitely more sophisticated than any petrol gauge. Even though most petrol gauges have the secondary warning of a flashing light, how many of us have never, ever run out of petrol? I don't suppose most of us would have survived our thirties if running out of petrol meant death.

Stop seeing hunger as an evil, but as the friend it truly is

It was this realization – that hunger is not an evil but an incredibly ingenious device to give us endless pleasure without suffering any consequent aggravation – that was the second of the important pieces of evidence which I referred to earlier. It only occurred to me when comparing the close association between craving for a cigarette and hunger for food. It was the most significant piece of evidence of all, in that it removed the belief I had that my method couldn't possibly work for eating habits, this block I had that it is easy to abstain completely, but impossible to cut down and control.

The beautiful truth is that it is even more effective for weight control – you don't have to abstain! You don't even have to cut down! You can go on enjoying satisfying your hunger for the rest of your life. Provided, of course, that you follow Mother Nature's guide and all of the instructions.

However, supposing you aren't allowed to relieve your hunger immediately, then hunger is terrible, isn't it? Just think. What actual pain do you suffer when you are hungry? OK, your stomach might be rumbling, but that's not physical pain. Any aggravation that you are suffering is purely psychological. Wild animals are meant to get into a panic if they are hungry. This is what ensures that they find food as quickly as possible. But we can use our intelligence to reverse the situation. If you start moping because you aren't allowed to satisfy your hunger immediately, then of course you will be miserable. But if you see the situation as it really is: the longer you go without food, the greater will be your appetite and the more enjoyable it will be when you eventually eat that meal, then even the delay in satisfying your hunger becomes a pleasure.

I have said that the foods which taste the best also happen to be the ones which are of greatest benefit to you. It is not possible to understand this without understanding

The important association between hunger and taste

17

THE IMPORTANT ASSOCIATION BETWEEN HUNGER AND TASTE

The French are widely considered to be the leading experts on the pleasures of eating. It is not a coincidence that, before a meal, they say 'Bon appétit' – not a wish that you eat good food, but that you have a good appetite. What does 'a good appetite' mean? Doesn't it really mean, **BOY AM I HUNGRY!**

The point I am making is that you cannot enjoy the taste of food unless you are hungry. You might find this hard to accept. Many people believe that food either tastes good or it doesn't. So let's test it out. What is your favourite food? Try eating not one, but many portions of your favourite food. You will not only be sick, but sick of the taste! In fact you don't even have to go through the experience yourself. Did you ever see the film *Cool Hand Luke* in which Paul Newman had to consume all those boiled eggs? I haven't eaten a boiled egg since. If you think back on your life, you can probably remember an occasion when you made yourself feel sick by eating too much rich food at one sitting.

If you love curries as I do, you will know how gorgeous they smell and taste when you are hungry. If you have eaten more than you should, you will also know that the same smell that was driving you crazy with anticipation a few minutes earlier, soon becomes decidedly offensive. Particularly if you are sitting near the kitchen and your nose is being bombarded with the smell of other peoples' curries. I once ate half a Chinese take-away in bed and woke up with the other half still in the bedroom. I didn't eat another Chinese meal for many months.

Food only tastes good if you are hungry. If you were to go long enough without food, even a rat would taste good. You might find that difficult to believe, but anyone who has been subjected to starvation knows the truth of it. We even stoop to cannibalism at such times. Fortunately, in Western society, most of us have never had to put the principle to the test. However, there are enough starving people on the planet to confirm the fact – that is, if they were lucky enough to catch a rat.

The film *Papillon* illustrates the point very adequately. The first bowl of gruel that Steve McQueen received on Devil's Island contained a live cockroach. He threw it out in disgust. We can all identify with his situation. We've all found something in our food that should not have been there on at least one occasion in our lives. Three months later, Steve McQueen was actually trying to catch cockroaches in order to eat them. Hard to imagine that we could be reduced to such a situation. You don't really need to imagine it – just rely on the evidence of people who have actually been in a similar situation.

Remember that the real pleasure in eating is in the satisfying of hunger. So the sixth instruction is:

Do not eat unless you are hungry

Food will only smell and taste good if you are hungry!

I'm aware that many of you will dispute this statement. Some will argue that there is immense pleasure to be gained from the ritual of eating. What nicer pastime is there than a meal out in pleasant surroundings, with a good atmosphere and convivial company? I agree with you that the ritual itself can be pleasant or otherwise. But that doesn't necessarily mean that you enjoy eating the food. I'm one of those people who, given the choice of pleasant company with bad food, or good food with lousy company, will opt for pleasant company every time. A meal out with friends is one of my favourite pastimes, but if I want to ensure that I eat a really tasty meal, I eat at home.

Because our brainwashed minds have confused ideas about the reasons why we eat, we try to clear our plates at each and every course of the meal. If you stick to the principle of eating when you are hungry and stopping when you have satisfied that hunger, you will not only enjoy every meal, but you will have no weight problems. However, I would emphasize that I said stop eating when you have satisfied your hunger, and not your gluttony. Does this still make you feel deprived? Just think about it. Is this really a restriction? Why would you even want to eat if you weren't hungry? Get it clearly into your mind:

Eating is pleasurable – over-eating is objectionable

I need to pause here. I can anticipate howls of protest. Am I another of these saintly characters that try to remove all the pleasure from life? Am I really trying to imply that there is no genuine pleasure in eating other than the ending of the sensation called hunger, that it's just like wearing tight shoes simply to have the pleasure of removing them? That is correct. But don't start getting depressed. This is strictly good news. In fact everything that I have to say to you is good news – remember the claim!

Wearing tight shoes can be decidedly unpleasant, but our Creator has so arranged hunger that we suffer no discomfort whatsoever whilst we are unaware of it, and can enjoy the genuine pleasure of relieving it several times a day for the rest of our lives. What's so bad about that? It is facts like this that make me believe that whatever intelligence or system created us intended us to enjoy life and that we only have ourselves to blame if we fail to do so.

The association between taste and hunger has an important bearing on our eating habits. Like most things in life, it's a two-edged sword. All creatures, including us, have their favourite food or foods, and while there are adequate supplies of those foods, there is no desire to deviate. Perhaps this is a good time to remove another fear commonly felt when contemplating altering eating habits – the fear that you will no longer be able to enjoy one of the great advantages that modern civilization has endowed us with:

The incredible variety of food

18

THE INCREDIBLE VARIETY
OF FOOD

One of the advantages of mankind's ingenuity is that, whether for smoking, drinking or eating, we have managed to provide an incredible variety of alternatives. Smokers have the choice of obtaining their nicotine through snuff, pipes, cigars, cigarettes, gum, patches or nasal sprays. Within those defined categories they have more choice, ranging from, say, five choices of brand of patch, to five thousand choices of brand of cigarette. Exactly the same situation applies to alcohol. There are literally thousands of different concoctions in which we can drink it.

We regard this great variety as very precious, yet it is a curious paradox that most smokers prefer to obtain their nicotine not only from the same category, but from the same brand within that category. This doesn't seem to bother them unduly. On the contrary, they tend to get upset when they are unable to obtain their usual brand. Drinkers also tend to have a favourite tipple. It's probably the misery we suffer when dieting that has ingrained into our minds the idea that this great variety of food is absolutely essential to our pleasure. But just as we tend to stick to our favourite tipple and our favourite brand of tobacco, aren't we the same with food?

This great variety is more apparent than real. Let me use myself as an example. Breakfast used to consist of a plate of cereal. But I would eat the same cereal day after day. Occasionally I might get fed up with one cereal and switch to another, and I would then eat the new one every day. There wasn't really much variety, but that didn't bother me. I think most of us are happy to keep eating our favourite foods. It's the same whether we have porridge, the great British breakfast or a Continental breakfast – we tend to eat the same thing day after day.

Even with other meals, the variation in practice is nothing like as great as we imagine. This dawned on me one evening whilst browsing through the menu at my favourite restaurant – the Motspur Park Tandoori. It's typical of Sod's Law that the best restaurant in the UK should be situated in a backwater like Motspur Park where nobody can find it.

The restaurant was busy on this particular evening. Joyce and I were prevaricating about what we were going to eat. Malik, the owner, started to reel off in a very matter-of-fact voice the particular delicacies that we were going to order. Obviously, it had dawned on him several curries ago that we always ordered the same thing. The truth didn't dawn on me until he began to do so! At the same time I realized that I did exactly the same thing at my favourite Chinese and Italian restaurants. I would laboriously plough through the menu and end up ordering exactly the same dishes every time.

Isn't it true that we have been indoctrinated to eat a variety of meals, partly to give us a balanced diet and partly for variety's sake, so that we don't get bored eating the same thing? Isn't it equally true that when we browse through a menu we are merely choosing the meal that we prefer to eat? In other words, we choose our favourite food. It is also true that our preference might be affected by many factors, like the weather, or how hungry we are, and our choice might vary from day to day or from year to year. There's nothing wrong with that. Equally, there is nothing wrong with eating your favourite food meal after meal after meal, provided of course that that food provides the energy and nutrients to keep you happy and healthy. In fact wouldn't you be rather stupid if you didn't eat your favourite food if it were available?

Perhaps you are worried that you would become bored with your favourite food if you ate it day after day. No problem – you can always switch if you want to, just as I would switch cereals occasionally. However, I suspect that one of the reasons why we eat such a wide variety of food is that we are not eating our favourite foods, we are eating junk food. The pet-food manufacturers keep coming up with concoctions that my cat will find unable to resist. I find that difficult to swallow. So does my cat. Yet for some strange reason she never seems to get bored with fresh mouse or sparrow.

So, once and for all, let's remove this block that EASY-WEIGH will restrict your choice. Just as today you eat the meals that you most enjoy, whether it be breakfast, lunch, dinner or supper, and whether you eat them at home or in a restaurant, so you will continue to eat the meals that you most enjoy. The only difference is that you will be eating meals that you genuinely enjoy and not meals which cost three times as much and which you've merely been brainwashed to believe you enjoy. You will also be eating meals that give you energy and *joie de vivre*, rather than meals that do the complete opposite!

This leads me to a very important aspect of EASYWEIGH:

The junk margin

19

THE JUNK MARGIN

Wild animals will always eat their favourite food, provided they can get it. But it's a fact of nature that their favourite food is not always available. If Mother Nature had programmed them not to eat unless they could obtain the food that was most beneficial to them, they would often starve. So nature incorporates this ingenious fail-safe device – the hungrier you get, the tastier second- or third-rate foods will appear, which ensures survival.

I said this is a two-edged sword. Let's use a gorilla as an example. A gorilla prefers to eat fruit. When fruit is not available it will eat other vegetation in order to survive. But it still doesn't become overweight or suffer from the many gastric diseases that human beings suffer from. This is good news for us. It means that Mother Nature has provided a liberal margin of error, and that provided the bulk of our food consists of the packages designed for us we can continue to consume large quantities of junk food without any harmful effects whatsoever. This 'junk margin' is a very important element of EASYWEIGH. It means that there are no rigid restrictions. You never have to say to yourself, 'I'm not allowed to eat this food or that food.' I'll be referring to this 'junk margin' in greater detail later.

I should explain that I use the expression 'junk' food, not in the context that a nutritionist would use it, but in the natural context. There are very few nutritionists that would describe milk or cheese as junk foods, but, as I will explain later, that's exactly what they are.

The danger of this margin of error is that, whereas gorillas and other wild animals will revert to their favourite foods as soon as they become available, Western civilization has reached such a stage that junk food becomes our normal diet practically as soon as we are weaned from our mother's breast.

It occurs to me that my frequent references to elephants, gorillas and other wild animals might have conjured up visions in your mind of Christmas dinner consisting of ripping off choice pieces of bark from your fruit trees. Not so. Fortunately mankind is ingenious. But from now on we are going to use our ingenuity, not to destroy ourselves by disguising junk food to appear as the real McCoy, but to enhance the real McCoy.

Earlier I referred to a paradox – *I'm already eating as much of my favourite foods as I want to and that's why I'm overweight. If I have to change my eating habits, I'll no longer be eating as much of my favourite foods as I want to*. I asked you to keep an open mind. Just as I asked you not to impede your efforts by fixing a target weight based on unsound facts, I'm now going to ask you not to decide your favourite foods in advance.

Now let's take a closer look at

Our favourite foods

20

OUR FAVOURITE FOODS

There is no doubt that Mother Nature's method of ensuring that we eat the food packages which are most beneficial to us is to make them taste good. However, we tend to think of taste as a matter of fact. Different foods either taste very good, or very bad, or somewhere in between. We happily accept that different individuals have different tastes. What I now want you to question is, why?

Do you think it is just coincidence that the Chinese prefer rice, the Italians prefer pasta and that before such foods became readily available in the UK we preferred bread and potatoes? Do you think it is coincidence that mother's cooking just happens to be the best? Or do you think that a more probable explanation is that we tend to acquire a taste for the most pleasant of the foods that are available?

Perhaps you believe that your favourite foods are not so much a question of choice but of taste. If a particular food tastes good you enjoy it, if it doesn't you don't. If certain foods either taste good or otherwise, why do our tastes vary throughout our lives? Why do we talk about an 'acquired' taste when referring to certain foods? How could you possibly acquire a taste if the food either tasted good or bad? If it tasted bad, why on earth would you want to acquire the taste?

There is no doubt that Mother Nature's guide intended us to eat the foods that taste the best. This is how it was meant to be. It is also obvious that Mother Nature intended us to 'acquire' a taste for inferior foods when the real McCoy wasn't available rather than starve. But there is no evidence that she intended us to stick with second best when the real McCoy was available, and I would suggest that your present favourite foods are not so much a question of choice or taste as of conditioning and brainwashing.

Let's test it out. If taste is a question of fact, why do our tastes change over the years? Can you remember the thrill of going to a birthday party when you were a child? Can you remember the brainwashing? 'You can't have any cake until you've eaten some sandwiches.' But what was the crowning delicacy after the sandwiches and the cake? Wasn't it the jelly?

Do you remember how exciting that jelly was when it wobbled on the plate? Do you remember the utter joy of actually being allowed to eat something so exciting? Oh, those happy childhood memories. Do you remember how cold it was? Do you remember how utterly tasteless it was? Jelly isn't expensive. How often do you eat jelly nowadays? I'm all for anything that can increase the pleasure in life, whether you are a five-year-old or a ninety-year-old, but by providing our children with jellies, and convincing them that a jelly is the *pièce de résistance*, don't we become part of the brainwashing?

Why are jellies one of our favourite foods as children? When did you last crave them? Why did my first Chinese meal and my first curry make me feel nauseous? Why, for so long, did they become my favourite foods? You must have met people who couldn't survive with less than four spoonfuls of sugar in their tea, and then cut out sugar completely – a week later, when you inadvertently put just half a teaspoonful in their cup, they spit it out over your best carpet as if you'd just given them a half-spoonful of arsenic.

This was the third of the three important pieces of evidence and is also the seventh instruction:

Don't be the slave of your taste-buds!

You will learn to enjoy the taste of any food that you regularly consume, so why not learn to enjoy the foods that are good for you, rather than the reverse?

Now perhaps you will find this concept difficult to accept. Some of you will be thinking that you've got to eat rabbit's food for the rest of your life. That isn't so. One of the beauties of EASYWEIGH is that there are no restrictions whatsoever, you can eat exactly what you like. But even if you did eat rabbit's food for the rest of your life, it wouldn't bother you, you'd be eating it because that would be your favourite food.

If taste is flexible, how do you know that I'm not trying to brainwash you into believing that the foods which are most beneficial to you actually taste the best? No! As I have already explained, taste is only flexible to enable you to survive. Taste *is* a question of fact. In due course, I will explain how intelligent man has fooled himself into believing that junk food tastes good.

The truth is that our eating habits are the culmination of an incredible hotchpotch of ignorance, misinformation, brainwashing and out-and-out stupidity that has little to do with choice or taste.

However, if the brainwashing has distorted our senses, how can we tell which foods really taste the best? The brainwashing and the incredible variety of food available in Western society make it very difficult. If the effect of the brainwashing has been to destroy our natural instincts, how can we possibly use them? But our natural instincts haven't been destroyed by the brainwashing, merely confused. Every smoker knows, before they light that first cigarette, that there is something evil and unnatural about smoking. The disgusting taste of the first cigarette doesn't destroy that image; on the contrary, it merely confirms it. But at the same time the addiction, combined with the massive brainwashing, confuses us and keeps us trapped.

It's exactly the same with our eating habits. Our natural instincts are still there, but they become confused by the brainwashing. You were already aware of most of the important points that I am making. You already knew that elephants are the most powerful land animals, that they are herbivores and that they don't need to eat flesh to obtain their massive bones and muscles. You already knew they don't need to drink milk or eat cheese to obtain sufficient calcium for their massive tusks. All I'm doing is trying to clear the confusion. That is the beauty of this method: once you clear away those cobwebs, it's plain common sense. I'm only telling you what you already instinctively know. Wild animals don't have these problems – we are merely going to use wild animals to confirm what we instinctively know! First, we need to understand why those instincts became confused in the first place.

Where did it go wrong?

21

WHERE DID IT GO WRONG?

Ever since life first appeared on the planet there has been a continual struggle between the various species, and between individuals within species, to obtain sufficient food to survive. Mother Nature has provided different species with various ingenious devices to enable them to survive periods of scarcity. Hibernation is a classic example, another is my squirrel who stored the nuts. One of the reasons for the success of insects like ants and bees is their ability to store foods.

The reason why the human species is the most successful on the planet is that we've used our superior intelligence and ingenuity not only to hunt, collect, grow and exploit an incredible variety of food, but to acquire the know-how to preserve and to store it.

However, there is one major set-back in storing foods. If you don't eat them other creatures will – namely, bacteria. We tend to regard bacteria as a rather frustrating nuisance. But they have just as much right to enjoy life on this planet as we do and, like us, one of their favourite pleasures is a good meal. In order to prevent bacteria from stealing our hard-earned food, we need first to preserve it. But just think what this really means: whether you cook it, refine it, freeze it, smoke it, pickle it, can it, bottle it, sweeten it, dry it or saturate it with salt, all you are doing is rendering it either unappetizing or inedible to bacteria.

If our food isn't good enough for bacteria, it certainly shouldn't be good enough for us! Any ancient mariner would tell you that, originally, preserved foods were essential short-term substitutes in order to survive a long sea voyage. But all mariners were aware that such foods were just substitutes, and made them susceptible to a variety of diseases (such as scurvy, rickets and yellow fever). They also made sure that they ate the real McCoy when they were able to go ashore.

However, as civilization progressed, as the population moved from the country into large towns and exploded out of all proportion, gradually the provision of our food transferred from the individual or family to huge vested conglomerates.

The majority of the population was often deprived of fresh fruit – it was a luxury. That was the reason for their debilitation. As the child of a working-class family, I clearly remember that my Christmas stocking contained at least one orange, a tangerine and some nuts. Like chicken, nuts were a luxury confined to Christmas.

It's rather sad that the broiler-house conglomerates and institutions like Kentucky Fried Chicken have turned chicken-eating into an all-year-round affair. Why has chicken become so popular lately? Could it be because of the bad publicity about eating red meat? Isn't it because we find it difficult to reverse the lifetime's brainwashing that we've been subjected to? Aren't we really saying, 'I accept that red meat is bad for me, so I'll compromise and eat white.' Isn't that really like saying, 'No way do I want to lose a leg, so I'll just settle for the loss of a few toes'?

We are now completely dependent upon supermarkets, freezers, packaged and processed foods. At the same time, we have been subjected from birth to massive publicity from these vested conglomerates, whether it be the Milk Marketing Board, the Meat Marketing Board or individual manufacturers of processed foods, not only brainwashing us into believing that these foods give us tremendous benefits, but implying that we cannot survive without them.

Let's just consider what happens when we process natural food. By far the most common form of processing is cooking. When you heat food above 125°F you virtually kill not only the bacteria, but all the nutrients. It becomes literally dead food. At the same time you make an equally disastrous change to its state. All foods contain differing levels of water. When you cook foods you also evaporate that precious liquid.

In the womb the baby's oxygen and life-giving nutrients are supplied purely by a liquid – its mother's blood. After it leaves the womb, for the first few months it is nourished and sustained purely by another liquid – its mother's milk. When we wean a baby, we talk about weaning it on to solids. From this point on we think in terms of eating solid food and drinking liquid. But we don't immediately switch the baby from mother's milk to steak and chips. The solid foods that we wean the baby on to initially are foods which still consist mainly of water, like mashed fruit and vegetables.

This high-liquid content is a vital principle of Mother Nature. That oak tree which I referred to in chapter eight obtains its immense power and strength from minerals and nutrients supplied entirely by water. Even man recognizes the advantages of liquidity. It's not just coincidence that petrol and the other materials with which we regularly maintain our cars are in a liquid form. This principle of liquidity and high-water content in our food remains important throughout our lives. Food with a low-water content is difficult to chew, to swallow and to digest, and it is difficult to assimilate the nutrients and dispose of the toxins and wastes. Think of the plastic bucket syndrome. The fact is that we can survive far longer without food than without water. So how much more valuable do you think a food is that has a high water content?

The real problem with our eating habits is that, instead of following the manufacturer's guide and consuming the natural food packages that our Creator designed for us, the bulk of the food that we consume is actually designed by mankind. Which is about as intelligent as letting a pet monkey design the type of fuel and maintenance materials you'd put in your car. It really isn't surprising that we have weight and other eating problems. Probably the highest accolade to the incredible sophistication of our bodies is that they manage to survive as long as they do.

So what are the food packages that are best suited to our digestive systems and also happen to taste the best? In spite of the generations of massive brainwashing, there is overwhelming and conclusive evidence to show which foods Mother Nature designed for us. Let's remove some of the cobwebs by first eliminating two important food groups that nature clearly did not intend us to eat. The first is

Meat

22

MEAT

For the purpose of EASYWEIGH. I use the term 'meat' to describe the flesh of all animals, birds and fish, including shellfish.

It is difficult to imagine anything more effective than the brainwashing involved in the consumption of meat. The fears impressed upon poor families – 'Are you getting enough meat in your diet?' The adverts that assail us constantly – British beef, Danish bacon, New Zealand lamb. The mere expressions we use – prime beef, best end of lamb.

Traditionally, we would wear our best clothes on Sundays, and the Sunday roast was the best meal of the week. What do we prepare for the most important meal of the year? The Christmas turkey, goose, duck or chicken.

Perhaps I'm making your mouth water. I sympathize with you. It's difficult to believe that the benefits you get from eating meat are virtually nil, and are far outweighed by the disadvantages. As for taste, there are few foods that taste more bland than meat. In fact, as far as the human species is concerned, it would be difficult to devise a food less suited for them than meat. Difficult to believe, but let's look at some undeniable facts.

We have already exploded the myth that you need to eat meat in order to obtain protein. The largest and strongest land animals are all herbivores. Ah! I hear you say, but who is king of the jungle? The lion, and lions are carnivores. More misleading folklore. A lion might be regarded as king of the jungle but is nowhere near as strong as an elephant and, in case your concept of a lion is a creature bursting with energy, bear in mind that a lion sleeps for twenty hours each day. An orang-utan, which does not eat meat, sleeps for only six, and any energy the lion does possess, it didn't obtain from eating meat.

It is true that lions are carnivores, but even lions prefer not to eat meat. Lions will kill leopards and cheetahs but do not usually eat them. A general rule of nature is that carnivores do not eat other carnivores. Next time you have an opportunity to see a nature programme depicting a lion or some other carnivore making a kill, notice that the dominant beast in the pride first rips open the stomach and eats the contents of the stomach. That's where a lion gets its protein from – from the vegetation eaten by herbivores.

After the contents of the stomach, the lion will opt for the organs such as the heart, liver, kidneys, intestines, lungs and brain. Apart from bones, meat is the last choice. In fact it is usually the creatures at the bottom of the pecking order like hyenas and vultures that end up with the meat. That is one of the reasons why they look so dried up and ugly.

It's hard to accept that we were not designed to eat meat. But use your common sense. If you were to try eating some raw meat, you wouldn't be able to finish chewing it, let alone digest it. Sometimes we can't chew it properly even when it has been cooked. We don't possess the necessary digestive systems and chemicals to digest meat, extract the nutrients and dispose of the wastes. It's true that the Japanese eat raw fish. But they have to marinate it, season it and cut it up into very small pieces in order to do so. Whether they enjoy eating it or not I cannot say, but the custom hasn't exactly spread throughout the world like wildfire.

Bear in mind that cooking food is a relatively recent innovation in the development of the human race and that it takes thousands of years for evolution to adjust our digestive processes to changed circumstances.

Meat provides virtually no energy. Fuel is built from carbohydrates. Meat contains very few carbohydrates. What's more, meat has virtually none of that all-important ingredient essential to good health and digestion: **FIBRE!**

When you eat meat, picture the animals that feed almost exclusively on it, like vultures, hyenas and crocodiles. A vulture doesn't really fly, it relies on thermals to stay aloft, and when it has gorged itself, it hardly has the energy to take off. A crocodile lies motionless either on land or in water for most of its life. Both creatures look dried-up and exceedingly ugly.

Perhaps you feel that the main purpose of cooking meat is to enhance its taste. If meat tastes so gorgeous when it has been cooked, why do we need to add seasoning or sauces? We add seasoning and sauces not to enhance the taste but either to give some spice to a bland taste or to disguise a foul taste. There are two important reasons why we cook meat. The most important is that we are incapable of eating it raw. The second is that it putrefies quickly and we need to kill dangerous bacteria. Even cold meats are pre-cooked. But cooking not only kills bacteria, it also kills many nutrients that are in food. The other great damage caused by cooking is that it evaporates the all-important moisture. Meat is already somewhat deficient in that essential ingredient even before it is cooked.

Another clue as to whether we were intended to eat

meat is our teeth. Carnivores have long incisors or fangs and long, sharp claws designed to tear flesh. They possess much more hydrochloric acid than humans. Hydrochloric acid is used to break down the toxins in meat. Meat putrefies quickly, so carnivores have comparatively short intestines designed to dispose of the decomposing meat in the shortest possible time.

We are not even emotionally equipped to eat meat. As Harvey Diamond says, 'Give a child an apple and a rabbit. If it eats the rabbit and plays with the apple, I'll buy you a new car.' Observe your pet cat. Cats are genuine carnivores – even thousands of years of domestication haven't changed their natural instincts. The slightest scratching noise will start their ears gyrating. Whether it be a bird, a mouse or a length of wool, a cat can no more resist pouncing on it than you could resist blinking if I tried to poke my finger in your eye. Its natural instinct is to kill and eat anything that moves.

Such behaviour is abhorrent to us. Imagine driving through the countryside in spring and spotting a newborn lamb gambolling about with the sheer joy of being alive. Are you overcome with some primeval urge to pounce on it, tear its throat out and gorge on the blood and gore? Or do you turn to your companion and say, 'Ah! Just look at that'?

Perhaps you feel that we are civilized human beings and have been educated not to commit such barbarous acts. In fact the exact reverse is the case. Those lambs are being bred solely so that we can slaughter them and eat them. There has been much publicity lately about the evils of raising battery hens and the veal trade. The rearing of animals, be they lambs, chickens, cows or pigs, is a highly organized commercial business which goes out of its way to make sure that our consciences aren't pricked and our appetites aren't ruined by having to see or even think about the gory details. Another part of the brainwashing is to give different names to dead meat. We don't eat cows, hens, deer, calves or pigs – but beef, chicken, venison, veal and pork.

The next time you order lamb, think of one of those little bundles of bouncing joy. Do you think you would have the stomach to kill it yourself? The truth is that most of us wouldn't eat meat if we had to kill the animals ourselves.

Perhaps you suspect that I'm preying on your conscience to persuade you not to eat meat for purely moral reasons. Not so, I'm merely pointing out that human beings are not natural carnivores. Not only do we not have the stomach to eat animals, we don't even have the heart or desire to do so. Our natural instinct is to love animals. We find the thought of eating our pets abhorrent, and the creatures that we have been taught to abhor, like rats, snakes and spiders, we cannot abide the thought of touching, let alone eating!

Do you keep your pets so that you can eat them if times get hard? I have no doubt that during times of scarcity man has resorted to eating his pets rather than watch his family starve, and this was probably the origin of today's highly organized meat industry. It is a fact that man has even resorted to cannibalism at such times. No matter how abhorrent I find such behaviour, I'm fortunate never to have suffered prolonged hunger, let alone starvation, and I therefore am not qualified to judge.

I know of several cases where people have reared chickens or pigs with the sole intention of eating them. Yet when it came to the crunch, not only did they not have the heart to kill the animals themselves, but they wouldn't allow anyone else to oblige.

Forget pets and domesticated animals. Most of us go out of our way to feed and protect wild animals. We love our gardens to be filled with a variety of birds and wildlife. We love animals. Any concerns we might have are that the animals are not being treated properly or are unhappy. When you visit a zoo are you admiring each creature, or are you, like Red Riding Hood's wolf, sizing each one up, licking your chops with a gleam in your eye and thinking, 'I really would love to eat you'? Yet when you see a plum tree laden with large, juicy, ripe plums, that is exactly what you think.

Man is superior to wild animals. That superiority confers a responsibility upon us. Wildlife depends upon us for protection of both itself and its environment. Do you not think there is anything wrong in rearing animals that have faith in us because we feed them, shelter them and protect them, and then to betray that faith by slaughtering them and eating them? Do you not think it ironic that we describe kindly behaviour as humane and unkind behaviour as beastly? Somehow we seem to have got it back to front!

Not only do we have an abhorrence about killing live animals ourselves, but most people find the sight of a living creature in the wild being slaughtered by a predator rather disconcerting. When your cat catches a fluffy blue tit, where do your sympathies lie? We can forgive such acts as part of nature with the excuse that the predator has a right to survive or knows no better. It's one thing killing animals in order to survive, but don't you think that there is something really sick and evil about rearing living creatures

Just to be able to slaughter them and eat them?

It would be excusable if we didn't already have an abundance of food and if we needed to do so in order to survive. But when meat makes us overweight, lethargic and unhealthy, has nothing going for it whatsoever and prevents us from eating the foods that would leave us bursting with health and energy,

It is nothing less than ignorance and stupidity!

However, the main argument against eating meat is not only that it provides a minimum of benefits, but that it is the most difficult food type to digest and from which to dispose of the wastes. Even when you've cooked it and chewed it, the human body does not possess the correct enzymes to digest meat. It provides no energy, yet uses maximum energy to digest.

Meat has a comparatively low water content to begin with and, because it has to be cooked before we can eat it, the bulk of the precious moisture it does have evaporates. Our stomachs find meat difficult to break down and it takes about twenty hours to pass through the thirty feet of intestinal tract. Meat creates a maximum of waste to dispose of.

Imagine spending an hour spreading your lawn with what you think is a fertilizer, discovering that it is in fact a lawn poison, then spending the whole of the following day trying to remove it. You'd be upset if you did that by accident. No way would you deliberately do it. It's hard to accept, but that is virtually what we are doing when we eat meat.

No doubt you think I'm exaggerating. That's partly

because you cannot see what happens inside your body when you eat meat, and partly because your body is capable of surviving the punishment – or, more accurately, because up to now you are still alive. But is that really a plausible excuse for treating your body like a waste-disposal unit? Unless you follow Mother Nature's guide, you need to start thinking about what's happening inside your body. The BSE scare is just one of many tragedies that can occur when animals are forced to eat foods that are not natural to them.

Let's face up to the indisputable facts – eating meat doesn't seem to have a lot going for it. Now, just as we can solve the problem of getting the bucket into our petrol tank by cutting it up, so we can solve the problem of chewing and digesting meat by cooking it. But in both cases, not only do we gain absolutely nothing, but we cause a lot of problems. Man with his intelligent brain has solved the problem of chewing meat, but wouldn't the really sensible solution be to heed the obvious warning signs that our manufacturer's guide has equipped us with, and not to eat meat – or at least, not so much of it?

Now let's take a look at another group of foods that we have been brainwashed to believe are not only nutritious but vital to our survival, but which are actually shortening our lives:

Milk and dairy products

23

MILK AND DAIRY PRODUCTS

DRINKA PINTA MILKA DAY! Anyone of my generation will remember that slogan. I don't think any of us can be blamed for believing the merit of it. Even today, when I know it is nonsense, when I'm thirsty I find my natural tendency is to reach for a pint of milk rather than a glass of water.

Is it really surprising? At infant school it was compulsory to drink milk whether you wanted to or not. The indoctrination was continued in secondary school. It's only in comparatively recent years that doctors have begun to be aware of the terrible damage that milk and other dairy products have been causing. Even then, they don't go the whole hog, but merely advise us to use skimmed milk or cut out the cream.

When I talk about milk and dairy products, I'm really talking about milk. Dairy products, whether they be cream, cheese, yoghurt or butter, are merely processed milk. Regard them as just that – processed milk.

I must confess that it is this aspect of the brainwashing which I've found the most difficult to counter. Surely the authorities wouldn't have made it compulsory to drink milk if it wasn't doing us a lot of good? No way would they insist upon it if it were actually doing us harm.

But, of course, in those days I was young and naïve. I really believed that an expert was just that – expert on a particular subject. I didn't realize that an expert was just someone who fully believed the latest misconceptions rather than those of the previous generation. Who was I to question their expertise when they stated their dicta with such confidence and authority, even when those dicta contradicted plain common sense?

It's not difficult to understand why we were fooled. After all, the favourite food of all newly born mammals is the food designed for them – milk from their mothers' breasts. What could be more natural? This is the reason why I found the consumption of milk the most difficult misconception to counter.

Just think of a healthy baby being suckled on its healthy mother's breast. Do we worry that it isn't eating a sufficiently varied diet? Do we try to shove vitamins, calcium or iron tablets down its throat? Of course we don't. We instinctively know that it is having the food that nature intended. We are using the manufacturer's guide and we know that the baby is receiving the correct package. Look at the incredible rate at which all mammals grow and prosper on that package. According to H. G. Wells, the food of the gods was royal honey. It might be for bees. But for mammals it is blatantly obvious that the food of the gods is mother's milk.

The more discerning of you will have noticed that I say not just milk, but mother's milk. Isn't it true that, provided the mother is healthy and is producing sufficient milk for her baby, she is confident that her baby is receiving the correct diet? Isn't it also true that the mother only begins to worry if she is feeding her baby bottled milk and that our dietary problems only begin when the baby has to be weaned? In other words, when we stop using Mother Nature's guide and start to rely on the baby-food conglomerates. No great problem here, because the conglomerates provide the natural foods that mothers would have provided before the conglomerates existed – mashed fruit and vegetables. However, the baby is now not only being weaned off milk, but off nature's guide. The brainwashing of human experts has commenced and with it come doubts and uncertainties.

So, if milk is the true food of the gods and the choice of Mother Nature, if milk alone can sustain a baby with all the nutrients it requires at the most stressful and vulnerable period of its life, how can I possibly knock it? What possible harm can there be in drinking large quantities of milk for the rest of our lives?

There are two sound and common-sense reasons why we should no longer drink milk. The first is that the package was designed specifically for a particular infant. So sophisticated is it that the nutrient content varies as the baby grows. One important point is that all baby mammals start life on a diet consisting of milk only. But there is no such thing as the definitive milk. It is a different concoction for each species. The milk of a seal is nectar to its offspring, but would be poison to a mouse.

The second important point is that Mother Nature designed milk for babies. She also planned that all mammals should be weaned off milk at a comparatively early age. Do you know of any adult animals, apart from human beings and domesticated pets, that actually drink milk?

Even cows don't drink milk!

Let's go back to our cars. The choke is an ingenious device which provides a richer mixture of air and petrol vapour to facilitate easy starting and running when the engine is cool. However, as the engine warms up the mixture gradually returns to the ideal for normal running. Prolonged running with the choke out will rapidly shorten the life of the engine. This might not be apparent to the driver himself, but the excess exhaust fumes make it blatantly obvious to the driver of the car behind.

If Mother Nature designed us to be weaned off milk, how can anyone who describes themself as intelligent contradict that law? The enzymes necessary to break down and digest milk are renin and lactase. They are all but gone by the age of three in most humans. Our bodies aren't designed to digest milk once we have been weaned and an enormous burden is imposed on your digestive and waste-disposal systems by continuing to drink milk after being weaned. You can go on drinking milk, but do you really want to? If so, bear in mind that all milk contains casein which coagulates in the stomach to form large, tough, dense curds which are difficult to digest. Cows' milk has 300 times more casein than human milk.

Why in this enlightened day is milk the only food product regularly delivered daily to our doorsteps? Society is gradually waking up. Many adults have ceased to drink milk and even exclude it from tea or coffee. However, it is difficult to avoid it completely. When you eat pastry, biscuits, yoghurt, batter, chocolate, ice-cream, pancakes, yorkshire pudding, cakes, cream soups or creamed potatoes, you are consuming milk.

It is blatantly obvious that adult human beings were not designed to drink milk, particularly cows' milk, or products derived from milk. It is even more obvious that we were not designed to eat meat. Neither were we designed to eat foods that have been processed by man. So what other main food categories are there? Fresh fruit, nuts, vegetables, wheat, rice, other grains and other vegetation. Perhaps you've considered that list and thought,

'Wait a minute, that would not only make me a vegetarian, but a vegan!'

Perhaps, as I once did, you find that a rather daunting prospect. I'm not a vegetarian, but I no longer have any worries or fears about the prospect that I might become one. If at this stage the thought that you might become a vegetarian causes you consternation, let me point out that the items listed already form the main part of most people's food intake. Perhaps this is also a good time to remind you of the claim. You can eat as much of your favourite foods as you want to, as often as you want to and be the exact weight that you want to be. I've mentioned that many people no longer take milk or sugar in their coffee. Perhaps this has given you the impression that you will no longer be allowed to have milk in your tea. Let me assure you that is not so. I emphasize that I will make no restrictions whatsoever. Remember that all-important 'junk margin'. All I'm trying to do at this stage is to open your mind. Not to accept without question what the so-called experts tell you, but to realize that there is a genuine expert that has already provided us with a completely reliable and authentic manufacturer's guide.

I said that I would make no suggestions about specific recipes. There is just one exception. The reason that I found the brainwashing about milk the hardest to counter was because, although I was aware that much of the food that I ate was junk food, I had always considered a bowl of cereal swimming in milk to be my staple health-giving food. True, even if the particular brand of cereal was already coated in sugar, I would sweeten the mixture with liberal quantities of sugar, and no doubt the sugary effect contributed a great deal to the pleasure of the meal. But if milk was taboo, it meant that I could never enjoy a bowl of cereal again. The thought of eating it dry was anathema. One of the most horrifying aspects of so many diets is having to eat dry biscuits. The thought of adding water seemed worse. If you like a bowl of cereal try adding fresh orange juice. It's absolutely scrumptious and you don't need to add any sweeteners.

Dieticians and nutritionists are forever emphasizing the need to cut down the intake of calories, but at the same time trying to ensure that we don't suffer from a deficiency of certain vital chemicals. As always, the intelligent human brain interferes with the laws of Mother Nature and comes up with completely the wrong answer. You don't have to worry about eating too many calories; calories are energy, you can't have too much energy.

However, if they are the wrong sort of calories, your digestive system isn't equipped to cope. That would be like the owner of a Ford Escort thinking, *A formula-one racing car can do over 200 miles an hour, so I'll use the same fuel*. It's the plastic bucket syndrome again. The problem is not that we consume too many calories, but that our digestive systems are not designed to assimilate the type of calories contained in some of the foods that we eat, such as refined sugar. You might find this difficult to understand, but would you dream of filling up your petrol tank with fuel designed for a jumbo jet?

In their desire to avoid vitamin and mineral deficiency, what doctors and nutritionists also tend to overlook is that it can be just as debilitating to supply the body with more chemicals than it needs. If you overfill your engine with oil, it overflows and makes a very sticky mess. But at least the surplus will run away. Overfill your body and the surplus cannot just run away, it has to be processed through the stomach, the intestines, the kidneys, the liver, the bladder and the bowels. In certain circumstances the body is unable to dispose of the surplus, and it then has to be stored. Now your body hasn't got huge warehouses in which to store these excesses, so it has to create its own warehouses – the rolls of fat that you have to carry around with you for the rest of your shortened life.

Imagine going to the supermarket and purchasing not just one week's supply of food, but two, then having to carry that baggage around, like a genie on your back, for the rest of your living days – never able to unload your burden for a single minute for the rest of your life, whether you were sleeping, working or relaxing. In Western society we don't have to worry about starvation now. Is it not more sensible to store those extra weeks' provisions in the fridge rather than carrying them around for the rest of your life?

Hard as it may be to accept that meat, milk and dairy products are not suitable for human digestion, it is impossible to dispute the overwhelming evidence. But what evidence is there to establish which food packages *were* designed for us?

You'll find the evidence even more conclusive. One useful clue is to find out what we used to eat before our instincts became distorted by our intelligence. To do this, we need to go back before cavemen, before we learned to control fire or to plant seeds or to domesticate animals. In fact we have to observe our closest ancestors.

What do gorillas eat?

24

WHAT DO GORILLAS EAT?

It is generally accepted that our nearest cousins are the great apes. You might well argue that sufficient time has elapsed since we left the trees for our digestive systems to have adjusted to our changed eating habits. Again, look at the facts – we are still remarkably similar in external appearance to the great apes, particularly if you remove the hair. Internally, we are virtually the same. It was reported recently that the DNA of a chimpanzee is 98 percent the same as that of a human being.

If they can get a sufficient supply, gorillas prefer to eat fresh fruit. If they can't get fresh fruit, they will supplement their diet with other vegetation. They never eat meat or dairy products. Some apes, such as chimpanzees, will occasionally eat meat, but the vast bulk of their diet consists of vegetation.

Before you start feeling sorry for gorillas, remember that they will always eat their favourite food provided it is available, and when you are next being indoctrinated by some so-called expert about whether your diet leaves you deficient of this or that vital chemical,

Think of that gorilla!

Ask yourself why he is so many times stronger than you are. Ask yourself why the human race managed to survive before it even discovered fire, let alone vitamins. Use your common sense:

Rely on the manufacturer's guide!

Perhaps you are wondering, *If gorillas are so strong, why are they in danger of extinction?* For the same reason that thousands of other species face extinction. Because if man doesn't destroy their environment, he pollutes it.

I'm suggesting that in attempting to establish the natural diet that Mother Nature intended for human beings, all the evidence points in one direction – **FRUIT!** That's what our closest ancestors, who haven't been affected by massive brainwashing, prefer to eat. If you look at the facts, it's what we prefer to eat!

Those jellies and ice-creams that we loved as children. What would they have tasted like if we hadn't flavoured them? They would have been completely tasteless. Did we flavour them with pork, beef, lamb or turkey? No, we flavoured them with strawberry, pineapple, vanilla. All extracted from fruits and other plants. And this precious meat that we treasure so much – we not only have to cook it in order to eat it, but if it tastes so great, why do we have to add salt, pepper, gravy, garlic, pickles and other sauces to make it taste good? Imagine needing to add those things to fresh, ripe fruit.

What do these sauces which we add to meat to make it taste good consist of ? We add apple sauce to pork, mint to lamb, cranberry to turkey, horse-radish or mustard to beef, sage-and-onion stuffing to chicken, pickles to cold meats – all extracted from fruits or other vegetation. Whether they be milkshakes, soft drinks or alcohol, what flavours do we add to our drinks to enhance their taste? Strawberry, raspberry, banana, orange, lemon, pineapple, blackcurrant, lime, etc.

We have been brainwashed to believe that we add sauces

and flavours to enhance the taste of meat. In truth, meat tastes bland or even foul without these sauces. If meat tastes so good, why do we need to alter its taste by adding sauces?

Do you know of a stronger seasoning than garlic? Why don't we need to add salt, pepper or garlic to fruit in order to enhance its flavour? If you add garlic to a dish, aren't you really tasting the garlic? Why do you need garlic if the food itself tastes good?

The value of fruit is indelibly recorded in our folk-lore: 'An apple a day keeps the doctor away'; 'They were so rich, they had fruit in the house when no one was ill.'

Remember the importance of a high liquid content in the digestion of foods, assimilation of nutrients and disposal of wastes. No food satisfies this criterion more than fresh fruit. Fruit hardly requires any breaking down. It passes almost immediately from the stomach to the intestines, and it is not until food reaches the intestines that the energy and nutrients can be extracted and assimilated by the body. This is why you'll see tennis players eating a banana between games.

Now you might well argue that if high water content is so important, and inferior man was intelligent enough to provide liquid petrol as fuel for the car, why wasn't Mother Nature intelligent enough to provide our food in a liquid form? She did! Fruit is mainly water. Many fruits consist of over 90 per cent water. This is one of the incredible ingenuities of Mother Nature – to provide what is essentially liquid in a solid form. Liquids tend to run away whereas solids are far easier to carry and to store. As an ancient Briton, would you really have wanted to trudge off to the nearest stream in order to top up the tank? Isn't it infinitely more convenient to plant seeds and grow fruit trees adjacent to your dwelling and let the trees extract the water and minerals that you need? These are then presented to you in food packages, brimming full of those vital nutrients, tasty and juicy, with which you can satisfy both your hunger and thirst at the same time. You can either do this immediately, or you can store them at your convenience for weeks. Don't knock the system. We tend to take it for granted, but the more you study it, the more miraculous it appears. Wonder in awe at the ingenuity of it, that Mother Nature doesn't require us to grovel in the earth to obtain those vital minerals. It's cool to eat fruit and fruit is very cooling to eat. Have you noticed that, even on the hottest of days, fresh fruit is not only refreshing but cool? Manufactured drinks will only be so if they have been refrigerated or if ice is added. Let's not knock the system but rejoice in its ingenuity!

The other beauty about fruit is that it contains little waste matter, and that which it does contain is easy to dispose of. When you eat fruit you obtain a maximum of energy and use only a small percentage of that energy in digestion, assimilation and disposal of wastes. Fruit gives you an energy surplus. Some people respond, 'Who wants an energy surplus?' Then they go on to complain that they are hyperactive, live on their nerves and find it difficult to relax, as if too much energy was the cause of these problems. You can't have *too* much energy, any more than you can have too much money. Energy is a marvellous commodity, absolutely essential for a full and enjoyable life.

Fresh fruit is the ideal package designed for the human species. Babies naturally love fruit; they have to be brainwashed into enjoying meat and dairy products.

Closely behind fresh fruit are fresh vegetables, nuts, seeds, grains, cereals and other vegetation.

In case you are worried about vitamin deficiency, these foods will provide all the vitamins and vital minerals that you require. As I said earlier, vitamin deficiency is one of the evils of civilized society.

Another great advantage of both fresh fruit and vegetables is that they are comparatively inexpensive, and if you possess a garden, they can even be free! Let's pause a moment to

Consider the implications

25

CONSIDER THE IMPLICATIONS

When you've considered all the evidence I hope it will be obvious that the ideal food package for the human species is fresh fruit, supplemented with nuts, vegetables, grain and certain other vegetation. Whether it be for energy, fibre, vitamins, minerals, high water content, ease of digestion, assimilation of energy and nutrients or disposal of toxins and wastes − fresh, ripe fruits are the ideal food packages for us. They also have pleasant flavours and are sweet and refreshing. The real clincher is that they require no additives. They are natural foods. **THEY ARE THE FOODS THAT MOTHER NATURE RECOMMENDS!**

You might well question why Mother Nature provided such a variety of fruit. Wouldn't it have been simpler if the Creator had just provided one package for each creature? It might have been simpler, but it would also have been incredibly boring. I, for one, am very grateful that such a wonderful selection exists. After all, variety is the spice of life − this is just more evidence that our Creator intended us to enjoy life.

If he had provided just one package, wouldn't we have objected vehemently? Isn't our real fear of becoming vegetarians not so much that we don't like fruit, but that we would feel deprived of a variety of other foods that we regard as precious?

We have already established that fresh fruit, nuts, vegetables, grain and certain other types of vegetation are the only foods that the human species can easily and effectively consume and digest in their natural state, without being tampered with by *intelligent* man. It's not only children that love fruit. All human beings instinctively love fruit. You might choose a chicken tikka as opposed to a bowl of delicious strawberries, a bunch of grapes, or a pineapple, melon, pear, juicy orange or whatever, but you have been brainwashed. A child will choose the fruit every time.

Ironically, even the establishment institutions that were responsible for the brainwashing in the first place are gradually being forced to accept the inevitable. Having been brought up to believe that foods like a prime beef steak and full, double, dairy cream are the tastiest and most beneficial, we are now advised not to eat too much meat, particularly red meat. So many people turn to chicken and skimmed milk thinking they get the best of both worlds. Everyone, even government officials who are usually the last to admit a change of heart, now advises us to eat more fresh fruit and vegetables.

Perhaps red meat is more harmful than white meat and obviously skimmed milk is less harmful than full-cream milk. But isn't that really like saying, 'Try to cut down on the arsenic or switch to strychnine, it's not so toxic.'

Why don't the authorities come right out and tell us that meat and dairy products are bad for us and that what we should be eating is fresh fruit, vegetables and nuts? Is it because they haven't the guts to do a U-turn and admit that they were wrong? Is it because of the massive financial vested interests that are involved? Is it because they find it difficult or impossible to believe that intelligent, civilized man got it so wrong?

Perhaps it's a combination of these factors. But before we start knocking the establishment, can you and I accept the full implications? After all, it's not that easy to do.

Just think of the thousands of years of research and experience that has gone into experimenting with different combinations of foods. Think of the thousands of cookery books. To accept fully what I am saying, you need to accept that the only result of all that knowledge and expertise was not to enhance the taste of the most succulent and nutritious foods, but to make junk food appear to be the real McCoy.

I must emphasize that, with the exception of the conglomerates like chocolate manufacturers who are fully aware of their intentions, the intention of all those home cooks, cordon bleu chefs and writers of cookery books was to enhance our food. Nevertheless, the result of their efforts was merely to persuade us to eat second best, either by devitalizing nutritious food or by dressing up junk food to appear like the real McCoy.

Now that's not an easy fact to accept. It takes both courage and imagination to accept this principle. Nevertheless, it is absolutely essential that you do. Beware of any food that is not in its natural state. In fact this is your eighth instruction:

Beware of processed foods!

26

BEWARE OF PROCESSED FOODS!

In order to reverse the brainwashing, it is essential to understand the full effects of eating processed foods.

Whether you cook it, refine it, freeze it, smoke it, pickle it, can it, bottle it, sweeten it, dry it or saturate it with salt or other additives, the processing of food usually has three very harmful effects. The first is to kill the nutrients. The second is to add toxins and the third is to reduce the all-important high-water content.

You might well deduce that this dehydration effect is countered when water or wine is used in the cooking process or drunk during the meal. Unfortunately it just doesn't work like that – this is plastic bucket thinking. Your body is designed to process food in the packages that nature has designed. In fact, drinking during a meal can merely add to your problems by washing the digestive juices from your stomach.

We tend to interpret hunger as a simple matter of our bodies saying, 'I need food!' In fact, hunger is much more sophisticated than that. Wild animals will crave different types of food according to which nutrients or chemicals are deficient. We tend to interpret the 'fancies' that pregnant women get as somewhat illogical. In fact, they are highly logical – their bodies are telling them that a supply of additional nutrients is required to accommodate the needs of the new life inside them and to accommodate their own changing needs.

This is another example of how much incredibly more sophisticated your body is than your car. With your car, fuel and maintenance materials are supplied through several different systems. With your body, the same food packages provide both energy and maintenance materials, and everything is processed via the same mouth and digestive system.

Your car is so inferior that it requires regular servicing by man. Different parts wear out at different times and need replacing. Even bearing in mind that all the parts of a car are capable of replacement, the life of the average modern car is less than fifteen years.

The human body is self-servicing throughout its life span. In spite of the fact that we treat it like a waste-disposal unit and poison it with tobacco, alcohol, car-exhaust fumes and other pollutants, the average heart ticks away for over seventy years without missing a beat. I wonder what that average would be if only we treated our bodies with the respect they deserve? Unfortunately, modern medicine has applied the replacement-part syndrome to our bodies too. Do you really believe that heart, lung and kidney transplants are the intelligent answer? Does it really need an Einstein to deduce that the only sensible answer is to avoid the cause of organ failure?

If food only tastes good when you are hungry, why is it that people who have gorged themselves continue to eat? They cannot possibly still be hungry, therefore the only possible explanation is that the food still tastes good. The true situation is the complete opposite. The food begins to taste sickly. We describe such people as gluttons or compulsive eaters, but in fact the gorger *is* still hungry.

How can that possibly be? How can you feel bloated and hungry at the same time? Because if you clog up the system with junk food you won't have provided the energy and nutrients that your body is crying out for. The point is, and I believe this is the whole key to EASYWEIGH, your body will go on sending signals to your brain until it gets the real fuel and chemicals that it needs. You might well feel bloated but you will still feel hungry.

Ironically, you will soon feel even more hungry or unsatisfied. It may surprise you to know that we use more energy in digesting, assimilating and disposing of our food than in any other single activity. We are not normally aware of this fact because once we swallow our food the process becomes automatic. This is why we get so tired after a big meal like Christmas lunch and need a nap afterwards.

So, if you fill your body with junk food, not only do you not obtain the energy and nutrients that you require, but you make the position twice as bad by using your already depleted reserves of energy and vital nutrients to dispose of the junk.

How do we solve the problem? By eating more junk! Not only does it not solve the problem, it exacerbates it. This is why people who are grossly overweight have to go on picking at food and gorging themselves:

They never satisfy their hunger!

The Christmas lunch is a classic example. We gorge ourselves on course after course, yet we still need more. The more junk food we eat, the more energy we need to digest and process it. Eventually, we are rescued only by the fact that we are physically incapable of eating another mouthful. But do we now feel fit and bursting with energy? On the contrary, all we want to do is to sleep and leave our bodies with the impossible task of digesting and disposing of all the junk. It's a completely fruitless exercise.

Ironic that I should have used the word fruitless. It is another indication of how important fruit is in our history and folklore.

It's possibly easier to see the analogy with thirst. Thirst is a signal from your body to your brain, saying, *I need water*. We rarely need to drink more than a glass of water in order to satisfy our thirst. However, if you try to satisfy your thirst with beer, you can drink two, three or more pints and still feel thirsty. That's because beer contains alcohol and alcohol, far from relieving your thirst, actually causes dehydration. The principle is exactly the same with eating. Eat the wrong foods and you will suffer from permanent hunger. You'll also suffer from permanent obesity, lethargy and ill-health.

It is important that you understand the reasoning behind the ninth instruction, which is:

Try to satisfy your hunger with real food – not junk

Note that I am not categoric about the last instruction – I use the words 'try to', rather than 'you must'. The reason, of course, is that all-important 'junk margin'. It's not too important to worry about this aspect initially. As I will explain later, as you progress through the programme you'll find that your desire to eat junk food will gradually disappear and it will become the exception rather than the rule. However, it is important to understand right from the start that you'll never satisfy your hunger unless you supply the energy and vitamins that your body is craving.

What would you think of someone who accepted a job paying £100 a week if their fares were £150 a week? That is virtually what we do when we gunge up our bodies with bulky junk food. We eat to obtain energy. When we eat bulky junk food we spend more energy in digesting and disposing of the junk than we obtain from it. That's why so many of us wake up feeling tired and lethargic instead of rested and bursting with energy.

Apart from imbibing powerful poisons like arsenic, you would think that the worst thing you could do to your body would be to eat bulky junk food. In fact, there is an even greater danger which modern man is regularly afflicted with:

Refined foods

27

REFINED FOODS

We enjoy eating fresh, ripe fruit partly because the flavour is pleasant, partly because it tastes sweet and partly because the high water content makes the nutrients easy to assimilate and at the same time quenches our thirst. We enjoy eating nuts because they also taste sweet. Hence the expression:

Sweet as a nut

In chapter nineteen I promised to explain how intelligent man deluded himself into believing that junk foods taste good. In fact I have already described one technique that we use to deceive our taste-buds and our natural instincts – adding fruit flavours to junk food. Another is to add refined sugar to junk food to make it taste sweet.

The process of refining sugar strips away practically every vestige of nutrition. Almost all fibre, vitamins and minerals are removed, leaving only the deadly remnant. Sugar makes people fat because it supplies only empty, low-quality calories and excessive carbohydrates that are converted to fat. When you eat foods high in sugar, because they taste sweet, you are deceiving your body into believing that it is receiving foods that are beneficial.

You could argue that sometimes even strawberries will be enhanced by the addition of sugar. Only if they are not ripe. Fruit is only meant to be eaten when ripe. By adding sugar to unripe fruit, you are not enhancing the taste of the fruit, but merely adding a fruit flavour to the sugar.

I have described why you can feel bloated yet still feel hungry. Eating foods that have been artificially sweetened is even worse. Not only have you not supplied the necessary energy and nutrients that your body requires, but you haven't even filled your stomach, so you not only still feel hungry but ravenous. How do we usually solve the problem? By eating more junk food. Do you solve it? Of course not! You merely make it worse.

The reason that we become overweight is not because we eat too much, but because we eat too much of the wrong foods. Your body, although it does its level best, is incapable of disposing of all the junk and toxins that you pour into it.

So, we now know the type of foods which are most beneficial to us and the type of foods which are most harmful to us. But before we attempt to undertake the practical business of adapting our eating habits, we must understand two other important principles:

Timing and combining

28

TIMING AND COMBINING

There is only one rule about timing – and that is not to eat fruit when your stomach contains other food. The reason for this rule will be apparent after we have discussed combining.

I had only ever considered the combination of different types of food from the point-of-view of whether their tastes were compatible. I was a typical waste-disposal-unit practitioner – my only duty was to ensure food tasted good. Once I had swallowed it, my responsibility was over.

Omnivores like goats are capable of digesting many different types of food. Yet rarely will they eat more than one type of food at the same meal. In addition to the problems we have created by processing our foods, our success in farming crops and animals and in preserving and storing such a great variety of food has created another serious problem – our tendency not only to eat a variety of foods at the same meal, but in the same mouthful.

Why should this create a problem? Because our digestive systems were not designed to cope with a variety of foods at the same meal. Now before you throw up your hands in disgust, this does not mean that you can only eat one type of food at any given meal. But you need to understand what happens inside your body when you eat incompatible combinations. Just as processing can turn nutritious food into junk, so can badly combined meals. In addition, badly combined meals increase the difficulties of digestion, assimilation and disposal.

A common example is to combine a high-protein food like meat with potatoes, which are mainly carbohydrate. The stomach produces acid-based juices in order to digest protein. The juices necessary to break down carbohydrates are alkaline. What happens if you mix alkaline with acid? They neutralize each other. The result is that neither the meat nor the potato can be digested. You have presented your stomach with an impossible task. The stomach produces more acids, which are neutralized by more alkalines. The result is stagnation, indigestion and heartburn.

While all this is happening, it is quite likely that other foods are entering the system, resulting in more chaos. I have explained why fruit is the package ideally suited to the human species. Unfortunately, when we do eat fruit, it tends to be as a dessert at the end of the meal. But if you eat fruit whilst other food remains undigested in the stomach it will not be able to pass on to the intestines. Not only will you lose the benefit, but it will become part of the rotting mass, and any nutrients that you might have obtained from it will be lost. When you next get heartburn or indigestion, try to imagine that seething mass of meat and vegetation inside your body. Badly combined food can remain in the stomach for over eight hours. Eventually, the stomach operates a fail-safe device. It says, 'Sorry, I've tried my best but there's nothing I can do.' It then passes the indigestible mass on to the intestines. There's not much the intestines can do either. Any nutrients that might have been in the food have been ruined. Any energy that might have been extracted has been used in trying to cope with a rotting, decaying, toxic mass that has then to be passed down the line and somehow disposed of.

I do not wish to be crude, but anyone who has suffered from constipation will be aware of the pain and damage it can cause to the bowels. The average time for food, other than fruit, to pass through the entire gastrointestinal tract is between twenty-five and thirty hours. When meat is eaten that time is more than doubled. Try to imagine the energy required and the additional strain on your system trying to force that matter and waste through your thirty feet of intestines. Let's enumerate

The guidelines for correct combining

29

THE GUIDELINES FOR CORRECT COMBINING

The following are the guidelines for correct combining:

1 Do not eat fruit with any other food.
2 Do not mix proteins with carbohydrates at the same meal.
3 Do not eat more than one concentrated food at a meal. Concentrated foods are foods other than fresh fruit and vegetables.
4 Non-starchy vegetables (high water content) can be digested by either acid or alkaline juices and can therefore be mixed with either proteins (meat, fish, fowl and dairy products) or with carbohydrates (wheat, bread, rice, pasta, potatoes, grains or cereals).

The other factor to consider is

Timing

There is only one rule on timing and that relates to fruit. Not only should you never eat fruit with any other type of food, but you should only eat fruit when your stomach is empty. This is why breakfast is the ideal time to eat fruit. Also allow at least thirty minutes to elapse after eating fruit before you eat any foods other than fruit.

From the above guidelines you might well be thinking, *But this means I can never eat fish and chips, or cheese with bread, egg on toast or cereals with milk!* No it doesn't! This is the beauty of EASYWEIGH. There are no restrictions whatsoever. The above principles are not rules or instructions, they are part of the manufacturer's guide. This isn't a diet. You are merely going to change your eating habits so that you can enjoy eating every meal. The whole object is to make the above principles your normal rule rather than the exception. There is no harm whatsoever in breaking the rule now and again. You can even partake in the normal Christmas blowout without gaining weight or suffering the inevitable guilty conscience that goes with it.

But the whole object of these principles is to pass food through your body obtaining the maximum nutrients and energy and with the minimum of effort so that you have sufficient energy to remove all the toxic wastes from your body, plus sufficient surplus to be bursting with energy. Never forget, the tastiest and most enjoyable meals just happen to be the ones that will provide you with the maximum of health and energy. Let's now consider

Beverages

30

BEVERAGES

Do you ever wish that it had been you that invented Monopoly or the Rubik's cube? What would you say was the marketing man's dream? With all these rich, overweight, calorie-conscious beings in the world today, just think how rich you would be if you could discover a drink that contained no calories whatsoever, yet tasted better than any other drink known to mankind and was a better thirst-quencher than any other known drink!

I'm afraid you've missed the boat. Monsieur Perrier realized what it was some years ago and many others have already cashed in on his discovery. He describes his product as 'Natural mineral water fortified with gas from the spring.' He doesn't say what spring or what type of gas. However, the water does sparkle like champagne. Ironically, M. Perrier and his competitors have to spend an awful lot of money advertising this ingenious product.

It's even more ironic that the real inventor produced the product over three billion years ago. It actually flows free out of every mountain stream. It's the drink that all other creatures use to quench their thirst. Until this most recent micro-second in the history of the human race, it was the only drink that humans drank once they were weaned.

However, humans had intelligence. This intelligence enabled them to improve on the product created by an intelligence a billion times greater than theirs. Ask any cricketer or rugby player what is the best drink to quench your thirst after a match, and nine times out of ten the answer will be a pint of bitter, or a pint of bitter shandy.

Now according to my dictionary, bitter denotes a harsh or unpalatable taste. That particular beer is named bitter because it tastes bitter. In fact I've yet to meet the man who, when he drank his first pint of beer, whether it was bitter, lager, mild, light ale, brown ale, stout or Guinness, wasn't secretly thinking – 'Have I really got to drink this muck? I'd much rather have a glass of lemonade.' However, it's only kids who drink lemonade, grown-up men drink beer! So is lemonade what we should be drinking? No. The belief that lemonade is good to drink is just the result of the brainwashing that we've been subjected to from childhood to adolescence.

So effective is the brainwashing that we've even been persuaded to drink beers that contain no alcohol. Just think of it: we teach our brains and bodies to become immune to the foul smell and taste, just so we can get the effects of being inebriated by alcohol. We then remove the alcohol and are left with just the foul smell and taste, then try to kid ourselves that we are enjoying it!

Whether it be food or drink, I'm merely illustrating how easily intelligent human beings can be conned. If we can be brainwashed into believing that we enjoy the taste of a drink that is named bitter purely because it tastes bitter, then how much more easily can we be hoodwinked into believing that drinks like coke taste good, even when the addictive cocaine has been excluded. In fact, so effective is this brainwashing that many of us think that a drink isn't worth drinking unless it is coloured green or purple, has a pound of fruit mixed with it and a little umbrella to protect it. If we saw our dog or cat drinking such a concoction, the sight would appear ludicrous to us.

I find it amazing that weight-conscious people will

decline cream on their dessert, yet happily devour cream of this or that soup before the meal and drink several glasses of liqueur consisting mainly of cream after it.

Ironic that M. Perrier and his competitors are having to spend so much money convincing us of what the manufacturer's guide has been telling us all along:

The most refreshing drink is cool, clear, water

Perhaps you still doubt that fact. Let's be objective. Just reflect back on your life and try to remember the times when you really enjoyed the taste of a drink. You might reply spontaneously, 'Well, I always enjoy a glass of wine with a meal.' So do I, but I can never remember draining that glass in two gulps, then immediately topping up and repeating the process. In fact, my pleasure in drinking wine with a meal is not so much in quenching my thirst, but more in feeling that the meal would be incomplete without the wine. I recognize that this is not so much a need as part of the brainwashing.

The times that I'm asking you to remember are those times when you were so thirsty that you downed a pint of whatever liquid plus another half pint within a few seconds. Doesn't thirst work on exactly the same principle as hunger? If you are really hungry, any food will taste good. Bear in mind that most drinks, including beer, consist mainly of water; if you are really thirsty, any cool, clear liquid hitting the back of your throat and quenching your thirst will taste gorgeous, whether it be beer, coke, lemonade or the refreshing and health-giving liquid that the Creator packaged specifically to meet your needs:

Cool, clear, oxygen-packed, cleansing, refreshing water

Perhaps you still find that difficult to accept. But imagine that you are stranded in the desert without water. The sun is beating down and your throat has been parched for hours. You really believe that you are going to die of thirst. What drink do you think you would be pining for? Suppose by some miracle you came across a plush hotel in the middle of an oasis. Lined up on the bar are pints of fizzy lemonade and coke, a pint of bitter with half an inch of gassy head on it, and a glass of cool, clear water. What do you think you would reach for? Perhaps you think your choice would be the beer. I used to think I would have opted for the lemonade. I now know better.

I once attempted to climb a mountain in Spain. I got trapped in jungle-like vegetation and believed that I would die of thirst. All I could think of was water. When I finally reached civilization, I had the choice of the usual drinks with which we tend to quench our thirst. I asked for water. It didn't matter to me whether it was cool or clear, I just needed water. Ironically, up to that time I couldn't remember the last time that I had drunk a glass of water.

Just as modern civilized man has brainwashed us to become almost completely dependent upon processed foods, so we have been similarly brainwashed to search for processed drinks. The authorities cannot even resist processing the water that pours out of our taps.

You might well argue that if they didn't process it we couldn't survive. Perhaps you are right. But isn't this another indictment against intelligent, civilized man? We've so polluted our natural streams that we can no longer drink out of them. But wild animals can.

No doubt this pollution and the questionable quality of tap water has contributed to our searching for other beverages. Equally, I have no doubt that the tremendous pressure exerted upon us by the authorities to continue to drink milk helped to establish this trend in our minds, and it's not surprising that powerful, commercial conglomerates with vested interests have been able to persuade us that their particular brand of drink is refreshing and will provide us with nutrients, health and energy.

We regard it as the most natural thing in the world to wake up to a cup of tea or coffee. There's nothing natural about it whatsoever. These are concoctions invented by mankind. Now, of course you'll enjoy a cup of tea or coffee when you wake up. They both consist mainly of water and what you are really enjoying is the quenching of the eight hours' thirst that accumulated while you slept.

The real attraction of both tea and coffee is that they contain an addictive drug called caffeine, and when the caffeine leaves your body you suffer an empty, insecure feeling that makes you want to consume more caffeine. The second cup isn't to quench your thirst, but to relieve the withdrawal symptoms created by the first cup. The third cup will be to relieve the symptoms created by the second and so on *ad infinitum*. There are many caffeine addicts who drink over twenty cups a day and cannot understand why they are permanently irritable and thirsty.

Incredibly, the coffee manufacturers have managed to pull the same trick as the non-alcoholic-beer merchants. It's unbelievable! Provided you are not thirsty, the only pleasure you get from drinking coffee is to relieve the withdrawal symptoms of caffeine. If you remove the caffeine, you remove the only reason for drinking coffee in the first place – and we think of ourselves as intelligent human beings?

OK, perhaps you are not so stupid as I'm making you out to be. Perhaps you drink non-alcoholic beers or decaffeinated coffee because you genuinely believe that you enjoy the taste of beer or coffee. Remember, I asked you to beware of any food for which you have to *acquire* the taste. That means it's really a poison. If you have to work hard to acquire the taste, it means it's also an addictive drug. Children and animals don't like the taste or smell of coffee, alcohol or nicotine until they become addicted. Even then they don't enjoy the taste, they only assume that they do, just as some heroin addicts actually believe they enjoy the ritual of sticking needles into their veins.

This is why as youngsters, in order to drink tea and coffee, we have to add milk and sugar to make it look good and block out the foul taste. As our weight problems increase, so we cut out the milk and sugar. If we persist, we discover in quite a short time that we can actually drink the tea or coffee without sugar. But if tea and coffee taste so marvellous, why can't we enjoy that wonderful taste the very first time that we omit the sugar? It's for exactly the same reason that smokers find their first cigarettes taste awful. It's because they do taste awful. So do coffee and tea. But if you persevere, your body will become immune to the foul smell and taste in order to get the drug.

Those of you who have not read my works on drug addiction might feel that it is well worth going through this learning process in order to get the benefits of that drug. I should point out that there are no benefits to drug addiction. I stress – I don't mean that the disadvantages of being dependent on a drug outweigh the advantages.

All drug addicts know that throughout their lives. What I mean is that even the advantages that addicts believe they receive from the drugs are illusory. In other words, there are no advantages whatsoever.

Smokers believe that smoking helps them to relax and concentrate and to relieve boredom and stress. In fact, it does the complete opposite. It's very difficult to convince smokers of that fact. But concentration and boredom are complete opposites – so are relaxation and stress. If you tried to sell the same smoker a magic pill that could achieve two totally opposite effects within hours of each other, he would have you locked up for being a charlatan. Yet that is exactly what smokers claim that smoking does for them.

This is a very complicated subject that is impossible to explain in a few words. If you need to understand it in greater detail, there is information at the end of this book which will enable you to obtain the necessary literature. The simplest way to describe it briefly is to try to imagine why heroin addicts believe they actually enjoy sticking needles into their veins.

We are led to believe that they sink to this level of degradation in order to achieve the marvellous 'highs' that heroin confers. Now look at it from another aspect. Imagine a heroin addict who is being deprived of his heroin. OK, perhaps he's a bit upset because he isn't allowed to have his high. But why is he getting into such a paddy? You and I like highs, but we don't get into a panic if we go a few days without one. Picture the panic and misery that the addict goes through when deprived of the drug. Picture the elation when he is finally allowed to sink that needle into his vein and end that awful craving. Non-heroin addicts don't get into that panic and neither did heroin addicts until they started taking the drug. Heroin doesn't relieve that panic feeling. On the contrary, it causes it. If you are, or ever have been, a smoker, you will be aware of the panic feeling of being without cigarettes. Non-smokers don't suffer that panic feeling and neither did smokers before they became addicted to nicotine. Nicotine doesn't relieve stress, it causes it.

Perhaps you think I am being over-dramatic by comparing heroin addiction with the occasional cup of tea or coffee. After all, millions of people consume tea and coffee all over the world without becoming addicted.

This is another common misconception. There is a widely held belief that many people can 'use' drugs without becoming addicts. The only difference between a drug user and an addict is that the former doesn't yet realize he is addicted. The only reason why you drink tea or coffee is that you are addicted to caffeine. Perhaps you still think you drink them because you enjoy the taste. But remember two of the instructions that I have given you. One was not to let your taste-buds control you. Another was to open your mind.

If it's easy to stop taking milk or sugar in your tea or coffee, then why not go one stage further – it's even easier to stop drinking tea or coffee. Then you don't have to teach yourself to cope with the foul taste.

During the interlude of one of my quit-smoking clinics, I asked, 'Would you like tea, coffee or a soft drink?' A woman replied, 'I'd like tea without milk, sugar or tea.' It took a few seconds for the penny to drop. What she actually ordered was a cup of hot water!

Perhaps you think that she was somewhat dim-witted or was just being facetious. In fact she was neither. Can you understand the psychology? She had been brainwashed to enjoy a nice cup of tea. But she was educated enough to exclude all the bad additives, namely the milk, the sugar and the tea. In her mind she was still enjoying a nice cuppa!

What she was actually enjoying was the beverage that Mother Nature had designed for us in the first place. Ironically, it was a particularly hot day and she would have enjoyed it far more if it had been cool rather than hot. But then, of course, she wouldn't have been drinking tea but plain, bland, boring, commonplace water.

We need to remove this brainwashing. We need to see these concoctions of mankind as they really are – mere confidence tricks designed to delude us into believing that man can improve on the genuine elixir provided to us free by an intelligence billions of times superior to that of mankind.

There is nothing more pathetic in my eyes than being at a social occasion and watching someone who has given up alcohol struggling to consume pineapple juice after pineapple juice in the belief that we cannot enjoy social occasions unless we continually pour some sort of liquid down our throats. Social occasions are enjoyable because you are relaxing and not having to work, because you are in pleasant company and are enjoying pleasant conversation. It is a myth that alcohol improves such situations. I cannot think of a single social occasion that I didn't enjoy when the company was pleasant. I can remember many social occasions that I didn't enjoy because the company was unpleasant, even though the drinks were flowing freely. The truth is that invariably the occasion was ruined *because* the drinks were flowing so freely, so that someone either became aggressive or was so inebriated that they became offensive and/or embarrassing.

So what are the drinks that the manufacturer's guide recommends? Water is the obvious one, that's what other creatures drink. If you feel it necessary to drink something else, pure fruit juice is best, but it should have no additives other than water. However, most fresh fruits have such a high water content that they can quench your thirst and satisfy your hunger at the same time. If you ate enough of them, you wouldn't actually need to drink at all. In fact, eating fruit can be a far more enjoyable method of quenching your thirst than drinking. At half time, footballers and rugby players will eat a slice of orange rather than have a drink. But if you do need to drink, there is only one logical elixir:

Cool, clear, oxygen-packed, cleansing, refreshing water

Just look at a magnificent, strong oak tree. If it can gain its size and strength purely from drinking water, just think what water can do for you! What we have to do is to reverse the brainwashing. But

How do we reverse the brainwashing?

31

HOW DO WE REVERSE THE BRAINWASHING?

The first step is to realize that you have been brainwashed. But this knowledge in itself will not solve the problem. The next step is to decide that you are going to do something about it. The third step **IS ACTUALLY TO DO IT!** And this is your tenth instruction:

Go for it!

It's no good just understanding the things that I say and nodding your head in agreement, you must make a conscious effort to do something about it!

Don't worry, I'll tell you what you have to do, and if you follow all the instructions, you'll not only find it easy, but actually enjoyable.

Removing the brainwashing involves a two-pronged attack. First, start seeing the foods that are good for you as they really are. When you next cut open a juicy, ripe orange or pineapple, relish that delicious flavour, appreciate that cool, high water content, visualize the ease and speed with which your body will be able to digest and absorb the precious energy and vital nutrients and be able to dispose of the wastes.

The second prong is to start seeing the foods that you have been brainwashed to believe are your favourites as they really are – mutton dressed up as lamb. A bad analogy, it should be pork dressed up as apple. Next time you eat a piece of meat, ask yourself whether the meat itself tastes so good and whether you really want to burden your body with the trauma of having to process it and dispose of the toxins and wastes for an energy loss without getting any benefits from it whatsoever! That's always assuming that your body is capable of completely disposing of those toxins and wastes.

Ironically, this is the aspect of EASYWEIGH that many people find most difficult to accept – the fear that they will no longer be allowed to eat their favourite foods. It's similar to the smoker's fear that he will never be able to enjoy a meal or answer the phone without a cigarette. And just as the smoker's fear is engendered by the willpower method of stopping, so much of the overweight person's fear is engendered by the misery suffered when dieting.

However, in my case I know part of my acceptance was caused by the realization that cooking food can ruin the nutrients, and that Mother Nature does not recommend that we cook food. I couldn't but agree with the concept, but because practically everything that I ate was cooked and, apart from a bowl of cereal, all my favourite foods were cooked, initially I found this concept difficult to live with.

I think this was because cooked food smells so gorgeous. You could well argue that one of the Creator's rules for testing whether a package is designed for us is whether it smells good. True, but that rule only applies to natural foods. Perfume smells great but you wouldn't drink it. I frequently get gorgeous smells coming up from the kitchen. I say to Joyce, 'That smells great! What is it?' 'Nothing, I'm just cleaning the oven.'

The main function of smell in nature is to enable us to know that food is actually available and to track it down.

We have already established that one of the ingenuities of hunger is that we are not even aware of it unless it becomes extreme, or unless some other event triggers off the awareness in our brains. A common trigger is the sight of food, another is the smell of food. Because we eat so much cooked food our brains associate the smell of cooking with hunger and eating, but that doesn't mean that what is cooking necessarily tastes good.

Smokers who are attempting to quit will enjoy the smell of other people's cigarettes, but if they smoke one themselves it tastes awful. We need to reverse the brainwashing that this association between the smell of cooking and feeling hungry creates. If you don't cook the food the smell won't tempt you and you'll find that you won't need to eat until you genuinely feel hungry. You'll then enjoy the food so much more.

Perhaps you think that what I am suggesting is a process of self-brainwashing. **ABSOLUTELY NOT!** This is a counter-brainwashing exercise and not nearly so difficult as you might imagine.

Let's use an analogy. Imagine you've fallen in love with someone with a beautiful face, perfect body, good character and with a pleasant personality and disposition. The problem is that, much as you are besotted by that person, he or she cannot stand the sight of you.

At the same time there is another person who worships the ground you walk on. The problem is that you see that person as ugly, boring and completely lacking in character, personality or humour. I'm a witchdoctor and you seek my help. I offer you the choice of two pills, each of which will solve your problem.

The first pill costs only ten pounds. If you take it you will fall in love with the ugly person and see that person exactly as you did the first. The second pill will cost you one thousand pounds, and when you take it the person whom you adore will reciprocate your love and worship you as you worship them. Assuming that money is no particular problem to you, which pill would you buy?

If we are honest I think most of us would buy the second pill. Yet, logically, both pills will solve our problem. In fact the first pill has two distinct advantages over the second: it is cheaper, and tidier in the respect that the second pill will leave the ugly person worshipping you without you being able to reciprocate that love.

So why would most of us opt for the second pill? I would suggest that it is because we would suspect that the first pill would merely trick us into believing that someone is beautiful when they are in fact ugly. I'm not a witchdoctor and such pills don't exist. But trickery does. Consider exactly the same hypothesis, except that you have been fooled into believing that the first person is beautiful and pleasant and that the second person is ugly and boring. After all, you must have seen films in which the star is made to appear plain and dowdy and then attractive and dynamic, or looks nineteen or ninety according to the movie-makers' desire. In fact you must have experienced many such occasions in your own life, when first appearances or impressions were ultimately reversed.

Supposing the reality was that the first person was the ugly duckling and the person that loved you was in fact the beautiful swan? Then you wouldn't need witchcraft or magic pills, all you would need to do is to open your eyes and your mind.

That is exactly the position you are in!

You've already been brainwashed!

The foods that you have been brainwashed into believing are beautiful, like meat, double cream, dairy products and exotic desserts, don't love you. On the contrary, they hate you, they are killing you! On the other hand, the foods that love you, sustain you and provide you with health and energy and that are good for you, you now take for granted and regard as second-rate. Vegetables are merely an appendage to the *main* course. Fruit is regarded merely as one of the options in a course which itself is treated as optional. We don't regard bread and potatoes as delicacies because they are relatively cheap, and we take them for granted at every meal. But since they are such a vital part of our diet, aren't they the real delicacy? After all, there are a thousand different fillings you can put in a sandwich, but the main constituent of any sandwich that you have ever enjoyed is bread!

The fact is that you have been brainwashed to believe that junk food is good for you. Now I assume you regard yourself as a reasonably intelligent person. If you can be persuaded that junk is good, just think how easy it should be to see junk as it really is and genuine food as it really is, provided you make the conscious effort to reverse the brainwashing.

The fact is that you won't be able to help yourself. You know instinctively that what I am saying is correct. Once you know the truth, there is no way that you can kid yourself otherwise. You'll find that from now on you will start to analyse all processed foods. You'll find yourself questioning the reason for the processing. Is it to make junk food appear palatable? Is it destroying natural food?

Let's use a classic example of a food that probably causes more frustration than any other:

Chocolate

32

CHOCOLATE

Practically every person that has weight problems says to me, 'I adore chocolate, can you stop me eating chocolate?' If they adore eating chocolate, why do they want me to stop them eating it? The obvious answer is that they blame their weight problem on the fact that they eat too much chocolate. If this is so, why don't they first ask me, 'Can you fix it so that I can eat as much chocolate as I want, without being overweight?' It's strange that not a single person has ever asked me that question.

I once had this problem with chocolate myself. I would open a box of assorted chocolates and pick out my favourite centres. The first one tasted gorgeous. The second not quite so good. From then on I would put chocolate after chocolate in my mouth and they would begin to taste sickly. I would not only devour all my favourite centres, but the ones that I wasn't particularly fond of. I'd soon be looking forward to the stage where I was left only with centres that I positively didn't like so that I could stop eating them. Amazingly, even when I reached that stage and was utterly sick of the taste and smell of chocolate, those chocolates would still be winking at me, and I wasn't free until I'd scoffed the lot. I didn't understand the problem. Now I do.

We were all brought up on chocolate bars and so are our children and grandchildren. That's why their teeth are rotting and why so many of them are so frustrated and agitated. Chocolate is made from cacao seeds. So is cocoa. Try eating unsweetened cocoa. It tastes foul. Remember, food that tastes foul spells danger. Chocolate consists of three basic components:

1 Cocoa, which contains an addictive, foul-tasting, poisonous drug, called theobromine. It's this addictive drug which makes you want to go on eating chocolate even after you are sick of the taste.
2 Refined sugar to cover up the foul taste.
3 Milk intended for calves to make it look pleasant.

All three components do absolutely nothing for the human body and cause differing levels of harm. However, their combined effect is to brainwash us into believing that we are consuming something pleasurable and nutritious. Chocolate is one of the worst examples of refined foods and one of the cleverest examples of brainwashing.

I believe that some people have this love—hate relationship with chocolate in exactly the same way that smokers do with cigarettes. Their instinct senses that they are hooked on something that is evil. Perhaps you think the addictive effect of chocolate is so great that you haven't the willpower to resist it? Not so. Addictive substances can only affect you if you take them. Avoid taking the first chocolate and you won't have to resist taking the next one. Would you eat excrement if it had an additive to make it taste and smell sweet plus a drug that made you want to go on eating it? You might well do if you weren't aware that it was excrement. But you wouldn't go on eating it if you were, no matter how sweet it tasted and no matter how addictive the drug. You need consciously to reverse the brainwashing about chocolate. Whenever you look at any chocolate, see the individual components mixed up into a sickly goo in order to con you. You'll soon be wondering how you could ever have been fooled by it. In *The Only Way to Stop Smoking Permanently* I described the ingenuity of commercial vested interests in packaging poisons to make them appear acceptable. Imagine enjoying a box of chocolates, then being informed that the centres consisted of a dead mouse that had been minced and flavoured. Do you think that you could have enjoyed eating those chocolates if you had known? Of course you couldn't. But while you weren't aware that the centres consisted of dead mouse, the refined sugar would have disguised the foul taste and you would actually have enjoyed them.

But theobromine is more harmful to you than eating a dead mouse. You need to open your mind and realize that these commercial conglomerates are merely dressing up junk as food. Next time you eat a chocolate, think about the centre. Believe that it is a dead mouse; after all, it might just as well be!

I've devoted a whole chapter to chocolate. However, chocolate is just one example of the ingenuity of mankind to brainwash us for commercial reasons into believing that a lethal concoction is food. There are literally thousands of similar concoctions and it is not within the scope of this book to list them all. In fact, the subject is already covered by the eighth instruction:

Beware of processed foods

The reason that I use chocolate as an example is that its consumption is so widespread. It is not only eaten in its pure state – forgive me for the contradiction, there is no such thing as pure chocolate – but chocolate is often used as an ingredient or covering for so many other concoctions which are themselves pure junk. So effective is the brain-washing that we actually regard chocolate as a flavour. If you want to taste the true flavour of chocolate, try eating cocoa without any additives.

Let us pause for a moment to see

Where we are at

WHERE WE ARE AT

Before we proceed further, let's consider what we have established so far. Using Mother Nature's guide as wild animals instinctively do, we now don't need to know what our ideal weight is any more than wild animals do. We'll keep our scales and weigh ourselves regularly and keep a permanent record of those weights purely as an incentive to prove that EASYWEIGH works. When we can stand naked in front of the mirror and feel happy with our shape, whatever our weight happens to be at that time will be our ideal weight.

We know what foods actually taste the best – fresh fruit, vegetables, nuts, wheat and other cereals. We also know that those are also the foods which are most suited to our digestive systems, enabling us to live long, healthy, and energetic lives. We also know which foods we should try to avoid – any processed foods, and especially meat and dairy products. We know when to eat – when we feel hungry – and when to stop eating – when we stop feeling hungry. In addition, we have a basic knowledge of the importance of correct timing and combining.

However, how do we go about the practical business of changing our eating habits to conform to those principles? How do we get into a suitable

Routine

ROUTINE

It's all very well for gorillas to roam around all day, picking a banana whenever they feel a little bit peckish, but most of us have to work during the day. This is no problem because the system is so flexible, not only in the variety of foods we can eat, but in the fact that hunger is so designed that for most of our lives we are not even aware of it.

Our problem is that we tend to let the tail wag the dog. We get into the routine of eating three meals a day and attempting to clear our plates at every course of every meal. In other words, the routine becomes the dominant factor. The type of food, volume of food and interval between meals tends to be controlled by our routines and habits. For the reasons that I've already explained, because we eat so much junk food we don't properly satisfy our hunger, so our routines tend to leave us permanently unsatisfied and overweight. If you eat the foods that are designed for you, you'll be able to eat as much of them as you want to and you still won't be overweight.

If you are a picker – one of those people that is permanently hungry and has to keep picking at food all day – perhaps you are worried that you'll still want to pick all day. Not so. When you switch to eating real food like fruit, you'll actually satisfy your hunger and will have neither need nor desire to keep picking.

But isn't routine just the same as habit? That was the problem before – we ate three square meals a day, whether we needed them or not. Yes, but the meals were not geared to our needs. On the contrary, they were geared to our destruction. There is nothing wrong with routines. Wild animals also have routines. Deer tend to browse all day, whereas lions tend to eat once a day. They do so for the selfish reason that it suits them. Fortunately, we can establish our routines for the same selfish reason. But instead of letting the tail wag the dog as we have been brainwashed to do, instead of our bodily needs and digestive systems having to fit in with our routines, we are now going to reverse the situation: we are going to make the type, quantity and frequency of meals satisfy our needs.

Remember, hunger is precious, you can only enjoy eating if you have a good appetite. You won't have a good appetite unless you feel hungry. You won't get hungry unless you abstain from eating for a period. Am I implying that you have to spend most of your life feeling hungry? No! As I've already explained, hunger is so sophisticated that, if you get into a sensible routine, you are not even aware of it until it's time to eat the next meal. Then you can have the immense pleasure of enjoying every meal as opposed to none of them. Even if you do become aware of your hunger and, for whatever reason, are not able to satisfy it immediately, there's no need to get into a panic, you still won't be suffering any physical pain. OK, your stomach might be rumbling, but there's no physical pain, and just remember that the longer that hunger lasts, the greater your appetite will be and the more enjoyable your next meal will be. As I said earlier, hunger is a precious gift – respect it, nurture it, treasure it. I believe one of the reasons why I enjoy my meals so much nowadays is that I only eat twice a day.

I strongly recommend that you commence the programme by making just one change to your present routine:

Eat fruit, and only fruit, for breakfast

35

EAT FRUIT, AND ONLY FRUIT, FOR BREAKFAST

By just eating fruit for breakfast, you will already have taken the biggest step that you will be required to take with EASYWEIGH.

It is hard for us to visualize fruit as being appetizing at breakfast. We've been programmed to eat fruit as a dessert. But this is just part of the brainwashing. Breakfast is the time when our stomachs are empty and the time when our bodies are most prepared to receive the mouth-watering, succulent, delicious, high-water-content, cleansing, health-and-energy-giving nutrition provided by fresh fruit. Most people find it difficult to believe that they can enjoy fresh fruit for breakfast, but after just a short period they begin to see a plate of egg, sausage and bacon not as the great British breakfast, but as what it really is:

A conglomeration of indigestible grease!

Some people worry initially about the lack of variety in eating only fruit for breakfast. This concern is completely without foundation. In fact the reverse is true. I have already explained that most of us stick to the same breakfast daily. I now eat four different types of fruit each day for breakfast and am quite happy to vary the choice between apples, pears, oranges, tangerines, bananas, melons, grapefruits, strawberries, raspberries, blackberries, plums, blackcurrants, redcurrants, gooseberries, mulberries, grapes, pineapples, peaches and apricots.

There are also endless varieties of each fruit. I have only mentioned a sample of the fruits normally eaten in Western society. Supermarkets now also stock varieties of exotic fruits such as mangoes and lychees. When you consider that you have a choice of these delicious fruits in an infinite number of combinations, the problem of variety doesn't exist. You can eat fresh fruit to your heart's content **AND YOU STILL WON'T PUT ON WEIGHT!**

Let me emphasize. I am not saying that you have to eat fruit for breakfast every day for the rest of your life. On holiday, I'll occasionally eat a kipper or some haddock, usually when I can't get fruit. But this is no problem. As I've already explained – the 'junk margin' allows for these digressions. Now:

What about other meals?

36

WHAT ABOUT OTHER MEALS?

I would recommend that you do not even attempt to change any other eating habits until you are completely content enjoying fruit for breakfast. Any change in your lifestyle involves physical, emotional and psychological adjustments. If you try to run before you can walk you'll end up doing neither. Even when that change is an improvement, like a better job or a better car, it can involve a short period of disorientation.

Just like with smoking, the only real problem is to reverse the lifetime's brainwashing. But it's not like quitting smoking. We don't need to smoke and, having established that fact, the easiest way is simply to stop doing it. However, we cannot stop eating and why should we even want to? Eating is both a necessity and a genuine pleasure that we can enjoy for the rest of our lives. Smokers find it relatively easy to change their brand. At first the new brand tastes weird but it soon becomes their favourite. That's all you need to do – gradually change your brands of food for those that are most beneficial to you. Remember, they are the ones that actually taste the best, and they will soon become your favourites.

One of the beauties of EASYWEIGH is that there is no need to rush it. This is your eleventh instruction:

Don't make a hassle of it

You cannot blow this programme. You solve your smoking problem the moment you cut off the supply of nicotine – you don't have to wait until all the gunge leaves your lungs before you start to enjoy life again. So you solve your weight problem the moment you commence EASYWEIGH. In fact, provided you follow the instructions, your weight problem was solved the moment you started to read it. You don't have to wait until you achieve your ideal weight. You start to improve the moment you take the first step.

If you make further changes before you have fully adjusted to eating fruit for breakfast, if you are still secretly craving bacon and eggs, you'll be just like smokers who quit by using willpower then spend the rest of their lives craving a cigarette. Any further changes in your eating habits would merely exacerbate the situation. They would have the same effect as dieting.

You will find that if you commence the programme by eating fruit, and only fruit, for breakfast, it might feel strange to begin with but, providing you use the counter-brainwashing techniques described above, after just a few days you'll wonder why you ever ate anything else for breakfast. At the same time you will lose weight, feel fitter and have more energy. But most important, you will enjoy eating fruit for breakfast. This will give you the confidence to realize that not only does the method make sense, but

It actually works!

This period also gives you the opportunity to apply counter-brainwashing techniques to processed foods like chocolate, dairy products and meat and to discover delicious, nutritious and beneficial foods to take their place. By then you'll be like a dog straining at the leash, ready to try them. Even then there is no need to rush. You'll find that you won't be able to help yourself. As the surplus pounds and unsightly lumps of fat begin to disappear, and as you begin to feel healthier and more energetic, so you'll find more and more that your favourite foods become natural foods with a high water content, and more and more processed food will appear to you as junk food.

You might be disappointed to learn that this book includes no recipes. Everyone that has vetted the book has made the point: how can you write a book about eating habits without including recipes? I confess that my logic agrees but my instinct says no. I believe the reason is that with every book that I have read about eating habits, I have found the recommended recipes to be disappointing. Rightly or wrongly, I had the feeling that I was dieting and felt deprived. With EASYWEIGH I don't get this feeling. In fact part of the excitement is making your own discoveries, such as when I discovered that pure orange juice on cornflakes tasted far better than milk and didn't need sugar added. I felt elation when I discovered that one of my favourite meals, bubble and squeak, tasted just as good without the meat, and that lamb chops, new potatoes and peas tasted just as good without the lamb chops. However, if you find that you need recipes, there are literally dozens of books from which to choose.

I think now is a good time to deal with a subject that gave me cause for concern and might be troubling you:

Must I become a vegetarian?

37

MUST I BECOME A VEGETARIAN?

A question I'm often asked is, 'Will I end up a vegetarian?' I know the feeling. I've nothing against animals but the thought of never being allowed to eat meat gives me a feeling of deprivation. There is no logical reason why I should feel deprived, because one of the beauties of this programme is that you can eat what you like.

My tastes have gradually changed and are continuing to do so. A few months ago I detested salads. Now my favourite meal is a delicious avocado, tomato, cucumber and lettuce sandwich. The point is that even if you did become a vegetarian, you'd only become one because that would be your favourite food!

For most of my life I regarded vegetarians in rather the same light as I did non-smokers and teetotallers. Whilst I admired their high moral principles and saintly ways, I found them a bit too holier-than-thou for my liking. It was quite a shock to learn that most people who don't smoke or drink abstain for the purely selfish reason that they enjoy life more not smoking or drinking. Much as I admire the principles of those vegetarians who are so because they find it morally wrong to kill animals when other foods are readily available, it was an even greater shock to learn that most are vegetarians for the purely selfish reason that they find a vegetarian diet healthier and more enjoyable.

However, one of the beauties of EASYWEIGH is that you never have to say, 'I'm not allowed to eat chocolates' – or milk, ice-cream, steak, cheese or whatever. Remember that all-important 'junk margin'. It is a fact that the human body, though a solid object, consists of 70 per cent water. Your objective is gradually to change your eating habits so that junk food becomes the exception rather than the rule, and your ultimate goal is to make at least 70 per cent of your total intake consist of fresh, high-water-content foods such as fruit and vegetables. Provided you combine sensibly, you can eat virtually what you want to make up the remainder without being overweight.

You might think that 70 per cent is a high proportion to reach. In fact it is not. If, like me, you only eat twice a day, you already achieve approximately 50 per cent by eating only fruit for breakfast. If you eat three times a day, you already achieve about 33 percent, and if you eat a salad for lunch you can then eat virtually what you like for dinner.

You will find anyway that a large proportion of your main meals already consists of vegetables. If so, the only adjustment you need to make is to ensure that if the vegetables are cooked, they are not overheated so that the nutrients are destroyed and the water content evaporates. One good solution is to stir fry or lightly steam vegetables.

You will also find that by applying the counter-brainwashing techniques I have described, as the pounds disappear and your health and energy level improve, your desire to eat junk food will decrease. I no longer drink milk, tea or coffee. I no longer eat sweets, desserts, chocolates, cakes, biscuits or dairy products other than butter, and a side benefit from not eating those things is that I now have no need or desire to consume refined sugar.

It took no conscious effort on my part to cut these things out. On the contrary, I obtained a marvellous feeling of security, pleasure and satisfaction when avoiding foods that I knew would contribute nothing and be difficult to digest, and replacing them with foods that I knew were beneficial to me. I found that I gradually lost my desire to eat junk food. I still use the 'junk margin' and eat meat and dairy products on certain occasions, usually when there is no suitable alternative available.

Quite apart from the realization that my digestive system isn't designed to cope with meat, I find that constant reports of diseases like mad cow disease and unnatural feeding techniques such as the inclusion of steroids in animals' feed, plus the colouring devices used to make meat look palatable, have also helped to diminish my desire to eat meat.

The only conscious effort I made was to eat fruit, and only fruit, for breakfast. Even that was no real effort. My only regret is that I didn't switch to fruit, and only fruit, for breakfast from the day I was weaned! To sum up, let's consider

A few useful pointers

38

A FEW USEFUL POINTERS

Wild animals eat when they are hungry and stop eating when they cease to be hungry. Human beings tend to eat out of habit, routine, or boredom, or because they have been brainwashed to believe that there is pleasure in eating purely for eating's sake. There are several positive steps you can take to correct these damaging tendencies.

Always be aware that the sole object of eating is to provide your body with the necessary fuel and nutrients to enable you to enjoy a long, healthy and energetic life. Remember that our Creator intended eating, or satisfying our hunger, to be a very pleasurable pastime, to be enjoyed again and again throughout our lives, and that the pleasure should be both physical and psychological.

Also remember that you will not enjoy any meal either physically or mentally unless you are hungry. Hunger is essential in order to obtain the maximum enjoyment from a meal. Arrange your eating routines to ensure that you are hungry when the meal is due and do not destroy that precious hunger by picking between meals.

Be constantly aware that you cannot satisfy your hunger with junk food. An easy way to stop eating junk food is to stop buying it.

Even today, it tends to be customary to pile up the family's or guests' plates with far more than they either need or desire. With one particular circle of friends it was the practice to provide a choice of exotic sweets and it became difficult to resist partaking of them for fear of causing offence. Whoever's turn it was next to entertain felt duty-bound to try to equal or even surpass the previous couple's efforts. Ironically, the main topic of conversation on these occasions was the unanimous desire to lose weight. No doubt at times when food used to be scarce such abundance was admirable. But times have changed. For the bulk of Western society our problem is that we eat too much food. It used to be considered funny to lace someone's drink with far more alcohol than they desired. Fortunately, the Don't Drink and Drive campaigns have enabled most sensible people to desist from this stupid practice. It is just as stupid to consider it good manners to force excess food on to people, whether or not they are overweight.

Remember, your family and your guests are as anxious as you are to lead an enjoyable, healthy life. They'll appreciate you much more if you assist them. If you find that similar practices exist within your circle of friends, talk it out with them: change the standards, make it clear that the good host is not the one who provides an abundance of expensive junk, but the one who provides a nutritious, beneficial, satisfying and enjoyable meal.

If your plate has been overloaded, either by yourself or someone else, don't feel duty bound to scoff the lot just because it's there or to be polite to your host. Personally I find it frustrating not to be able to clear the plate, but I now find it quite simple during the course to ask myself, 'Are you really enjoying this now?' If the answer is no, I stop eating. Remember, the less you eat at one meal, the more you'll enjoy the next.

Avoid the peanut trap. The peanut trap is the infuriating practice that friends and restaurateurs have of plonking down a bowl of peanuts, crisps or other tit-bits the moment you enter the premises. You've no doubt heard the expression, 'You have to be cruel to be kind.' These people are doing the complete opposite – they are being kind to be cruel. All they do is to put temptation in your way. If you can avoid eating one nut or one crisp you'll be fine, but eat just one teeny weeny nut and before you know it you will have polished off the whole bowlful. You ruin a perfectly good appetite and then wonder why the main meal didn't taste as good as it usually does. It takes no willpower for me to resist the temptation of eating that first peanut or crisp. I can't tell you the immense pleasure I get knowing that had I taken it I would have had to scoff the rest of the bowlful. The pleasure is heightened by watching the other poor souls shovel mouthful after mouthful into their waste-disposal units. Friends and restaurateurs need to be aware that they do their guests and customers no favours by providing such temptations.

Be wary of all processed foods. If you are particularly enjoying the taste of a food, ask yourself what it is that you are actually enjoying. If it is a sweet, exotic dessert, or meat covered with a sweet sauce, ask yourself if you are actually enjoying the taste of the food or the sweet taste of refined sugar. If it's the latter, you are being conned. I know many people that you couldn't force to drink half a glassful of cream or half a glassful of neat whisky, but mix the two together and they'll drink glass after glass of a certain famous liqueur.

Don't be controlled by the brainwashing or by your present taste-buds. Remember, high-water-content foods actually taste the best, and try to follow the rules for correct timing and combining.

Before concluding, I promised to deal with a subject which really has nothing to do with weight control. I deal with it as a completely separate subject because I believe it, too, is essential in order to lead a happy, healthy and enjoyable life:

Exercise

39

EXERCISE

Most dietary experts insist that in order to lose weight it is essential to exercise. It seems logical, but as I have already explained, you don't increase or reduce the basic weight of your car by burning more fuel, all you do is to shorten the intervals between needing to top up. Exercising makes you feel more hungry and thirsty, so that you eat and drink more.

You don't see snails and tortoises rushing about all over the place, but they aren't overweight. In fact, the human species and the animals that it domesticates are the only creatures that find it necessary to take exercise purely for its own sake.

If you undertake a course of exercise in order to lose weight, not only will you not achieve your goal, but it will have the same effect as going on a diet. You will regard that exercise as some form of penance and you will have to use willpower and discipline to maintain it. It is true that in the early days you will have that wonderful holier-than-thou feeling, but when your supply of willpower begins to run low and some other event in your life becomes more important, the exercise will lapse. If you don't believe me, check the articles-for-sale column in your local paper. You'll find more ads for exercise bicycles, rowing machines and other exercise gimmicks than all the other ads combined. Do you think that's because the owners have reached the peak of condition and no longer need to exercise or because after two weeks the owners got fed up with using them?

Nevertheless, I am going to recommend that you exercise regularly, not because it helps you to reduce weight, but purely for the selfish reason that if you feel fit and healthy and if your body is properly toned up, you will enjoy life so much more.

In any event, as your weight drops and your energy level increases, you'll find a natural desire to enjoy the benefits of being more active.

A word of warning. If you are not fit at the moment, start gradually. You will find that as your energy and fitness levels improve, you will automatically want to exercise more, and so set off a marvellous cause-and-effect reaction that will soon have you feeling young again. Never over-extend yourself. Your body and a little common sense will be sufficient to guide you. If you are in doubt, first consult your doctor.

Once you are fit enough to undertake hard exercise, you will experience the wonderful feeling of the adrenalin flowing. That's a true high. It will shortly be followed by two other marvellous situations. One is the pleasure of relaxation after extensive activity. The other is being able to satisfy that ravenous appetite and thirst without putting on weight and without the slightest feeling of guilt.

There are many exercise gadgets on the market nowadays, together with health clubs, videos, etc., all designed to help you lose weight and feel fitter and healthier. My advice is to ignore them all. Just as having to exercise to lose weight creates a feeling of penance, so does exercising in order to feel fit and healthy.

Exercise doesn't need to be a chore. Did we need to force ourselves to exercise as children? As a youngster, did you pay good money to swim, or go dancing, or play tennis or golf because you wanted to lose weight and feel fit? Of course you didn't. You did it for sheer pleasure. Perhaps you feel that it was only a pleasure in those days because you had the energy to enjoy such pastimes. You may be right. But that isn't because energy is limited to youth. It's because of the lifestyle that most of us have drifted into.

However, we are going to change all that, it's what EASYWEIGH is all about. If you follow the instructions you will soon be bursting with energy, and you are lucky in that there is a huge selection of activities to choose from depending on your age, strength, health and individual taste: golf, bowling, squash, tennis, badminton, athletics, hiking, trekking, cycling, skating, football, cricket, rugby, swimming, hockey, basketball, netball, skiing, gymnastics, to name but a few.

These sports can not only be enjoyable in their own right, but provide the additional benefits of social intercourse, creating a healthy appetite and allowing you not only to enjoy your meals, but to eat more and more often without becoming overweight. They also tone up your muscles and keep you fit and healthy. They add purpose and enjoyment to your life. There is an additional major advantage which is not always obvious. They help to remove boredom, which is in itself a major cause of overeating.

Most wild animals obtain daily exercise in the natural process of hunting or searching for their food and by avoiding becoming a meal for other animals. Western civilized man has used his brain to remove the need for either activity. Some of us replace that exercise with manual work. I am convinced that regular physical exercise is essential to enjoy life. Our bodies were designed to exercise and not to stagnate. Exercise doesn't need to be a penance.

It should be a pleasure in its own right and at the same time accrue marvellous additional benefits.

In fact, this is what this whole book is about. We've all received the greatest gift imaginable – the gift of life. As human beings we are doubly privileged to be equipped with the most sophisticated survival machine on the planet. If you were lucky enough to be born free of serious physical and mental defects you are indeed super-privileged.

We're nearly there now; all we have left is the

Conclusion

40

CONCLUSION

The title of this book might tend to give you the impression that the main object of EASYWEIGH is weight control. You would be wrong. Just as a book on stopping smoking tends to create fear and even panic in the minds of smokers, so a book on losing weight can have the same effect on the overweight.

The incredible success that my stop-smoking method achieves is because my prime objective is not to make smokers quit but to make them realize that they are going to enjoy social occasions more and be better able to handle stress as non-smokers. In other words, the prime object is to enable them to enjoy life. You might well ask what the difference is. The difference is both subtle and vital. If a smoker concentrates on giving up smoking, that smoker's mental attitude will be one of sacrifice and deprivation, resulting in depression and almost certain failure. However, if the smoker can first be made to realize that in fact there is nothing to give up and that he won't miss smoking but will enjoy life more, that smoker ceases to see the cigarette as some sort of crutch or pleasure. There is no consequent feeling of sacrifice or depression. On the contrary, the ex-smoker sees quitting in its true light – the ending of a disease – and the process becomes easy and enjoyable rather than impossible and depressing.

Exactly the same principle applies to weight control. To most overweight people this conjures up the same feelings of sacrifice and depression. Your third instruction was to start off with a feeling of excitement and elation.

If you were able to do that at that stage, so much the better. If not, it is absolutely essential that you have this feeling of excitement and elation now.

The main object of this book is for you to enjoy life and live it to the full. There is no need for you to be depressed or miserable. There is nothing bad happening.

There is something marvellous happening!

You cannot enjoy life if you are suffering from shortage of breath, lack of energy, lack of self-respect, dyspepsia, constipation, diarrhoea, indigestion, heartburn, ulcers, irritable bowels, high blood pressure, cholesterol and diseases of the heart, arteries, veins, stomach, intestines, kidneys and liver, to name but a few.

You cannot enjoy life if you feel at one and the same time guilty because you eat too much and deprived because you are not allowed to eat as much as you want to. Why not eat as much of your favourite foods as you want to, as often as you want to and be the exact weight that you want to be, without suffering from any of the above disabilities and at the same time be able to enjoy every meal?

It's easy – over 99.99 percent of the creatures on this planet do exactly that. They do it because they follow Mother Nature's guide. EASYWEIGH has explained exactly how and why that guide cannot fail to work. All you have to do is to use your common sense. You have a simple choice to make. You can continue to let your intake be dominated by foods that will cause obesity, lethargy, poor health, guilt and depression, or you can let it be dominated by foods that will do none of these things. But what they will provide you with is an abundance of health, energy, and *joie de vivre*, and the really big bonus is

They taste so much better!

What have you got to lose? Absolutely nothing! On the contrary, you have so much to gain. You too can:

Eat as much of your favourite foods as you want to as often as you want to

Be the weight you want to be

Enjoy an abundance of health and energy
and
Enjoy every day to the full

All you have to do is

Follow all the instructions

Why not just remind yourself of them now. The Appendix lists the eleven instructions together with a brief explanation where necessary. If you need a more detailed explanation, return to the text.

Enjoy life!

APPENDIX

Instructions

Message to Readers from Allen Carr

'I believe that Easyweigh offers a simple means of leading a fitter, healthier, happier and more enjoyable life. The pleasure I get from enjoying those benefits is matched by the pleasure I feel every time I hear of someone else who has succeeded in sharing that enjoyment. I welcome feedback from my readers. Please send your comments, whether they be positive or negative, to: Allen Carr, 1C Amity Grove, London SW20 0LQ. If you wish to receive a reply, please enclose a stamped, addressed envelope. Thank you.'

Thousands of smokers have become happy non-smokers easily and painlessly by attending one of Allen Carr's clinics, where with a success rate of over 90 per cent he guarantees you will find it easy to stop or get your money back. Weight-control sessions based on EASYWEIGH and offering practical assistance in its implementation are now also available at a selection of these clinics. All correspondence and enquiries about ALLEN CARR'S BOOKS, VIDEOS, AUDIO TAPES AND CD-ROMS should be addressed to the London Clinic.

STOP SMOKING HELPLINE: 0891 664401

Allen Carr's helpline provides 24-hour assistance to any smoker having problems. It is introduced by Sir Anthony Hopkins and Allen Carr himself gives the advice. The menu-driven system allows callers to choose categories according to the particular problem experienced.

ALLEN CARR'S CLINICS

With a success rate of over 90% Allen Carr guarantees you will find it easy to stop at his clinics or your money back

ALLEN CARR UK
Helpline: 0906 604 0220
Website: www.allencarrs
  easyway.com

LONDON
1C Amity Grove
Raynes Park
London SW20 0LQ
Tel. & Fax: 020 8944 7761
Therapists: John Dicey, Sue
  Bolshaw, Crispin Hay,
  Colleen Dwyer
E-mail: postmaster@
  allencarr.demon.co.uk

BIRMINGHAM
415 Hagley Road West
Quinton
Birmingham B32 2AD
Tel. & Fax: 0121 423 1227
Therapist: John Dicey
E-mail: postmaster@
  allencarr.demon.co.uk

BOURNEMOUTH &
  SOUTHAMPTON
Tel.: 01425 272757
Therapist: John Dicey,
  Colleen Dwyer

BRISTOL & SWINDON
Tel.: 0117 908 1106
Therapist: Charles
  Holdsworth-Hunt

BRIGHTON
Tel.: 01425 272757
Therapists: John Dicey,
  Colleen Dwyer

EDINBURGH
48 Eastfield
Joppa
Edinburgh EH15 2PN
Tel.: 0131 660 6688
Fax: 0131 660 3203
Therapist: Derek McGuff
E-mail: easyway@clara.co.uk

GLASGOW
Tel.: 0131 466 2268
Therapist: Joe Bergin
E-mail: bergin@
  napieruni.fsnet.co.uk

KENT
Clinics held:
Canterbury
Maidstone
Whitstable
Tel.: 01622 832 554
Therapist: Angela Jouanneau
  (smoking and weight)
E-mail: easywaykent@
  yahoo.co.uk

MANCHESTER
14 The Circuit
Alderley Edge
Manchester SK9 7LT

Tel.: 01625 590 994
Fax: 01625 590 989
Therapist: Rob Groves
Therapist: Eva Groves (weight)
E-mail: stopsmoking@
  easywaymanchester.co.uk
Website: www.easyway
  manchester.co.uk

NORTH EAST
10 Dale Terrace
Dalton-le-Dale
Seaham
County Durham SR7 8QP
Tel. & Fax: 0191 581 0449
Therapist: Tony Attrill

READING
Tel.: 01425 272757
Therapists: John Dicey,
  Colleen Dwyer

YORKSHIRE
Clinics held in Leeds
Tel.: 0700 900 0305 or
  01423 525556
Fax: 01423 523320
Mobile: 07931 597 588
Therapist: Diana Evans
E-mail: diana_york@
  yahoo.co.uk
Website: www.dianaevans.
  co.uk

ALLEN CARR
REPUBLIC OF IRELAND

DUBLIN
44 Beverly Heights
Knocklyon
Dublin 16

Tel.: 01 494 1644
Fax: 01 495 2757
Therapist: Brenda Sweeney
E-mail: seansw@iol.ie

MUNSTER
Tel. and Fax: 056 54911
Therapist: Catherine Power
  Hernandez
E-mail: powerhernandez@
  eircom.net

CONNAUGHT
Tel. and Fax: 094 67925
Therapist: Pat Melody Dunne

ALLEN CARR
AUSTRALIA

MELBOURNE
148 Central Road
Nunawading
Victoria 3131
Tel. & Fax: 03 9894 8866
Therapist: Trudy Ward
E-mail: tw.easyway@
  bigpond.com

ALLEN CARR AUSTRIA
Website: www.allen-carr.at
SESSIONS ALL OVER
  AUSTRIA
Free line telephone for
  Information and Booking:
Tel.: 0800 RAUCHEN (0800
  7282436)
Sonnenring 21
A-8724 Spielberg
Tel.: 00 43 3512 44755
Fax: 00 43 3512 44768

Therapists: Erich Kellermann
and team
E-mail: info@allen-carr.at

ALLEN CARR BELGIUM

Website: www.allencarr.be

ANTWERP
Koningen Astridplein 27
B-9150 Bazel
Tel.: 03 281 6255
Fax: 03 744 0608
Therapist: Dirk Nielandt
E-mail: easyway@online.be
Therapist: Valerie Popowski
Tel.: 03 288 8082
E-mail: poppyval@iway.be

ALLEN CARR CANADA

VANCOUVER
412–2150 W. Broadway
Vancouver, B.C. V6K 4L9
Tel.: 604 737 1113
Fax: 604 737 1116
Mobile: 604 785 1717
Therapist: Damian O'Hara
E-mail: damiano@telus.net

TORONTO
Suite 700
2 Bloor Street West
Toronto ON. M4W 3R1
Tel.: 416 737 9683
E-mail: damiano@telus.net

ALLEN CARR CARIBBEAN

11 Lot du Moulin
97190 Gosier

Guadeloupe
Antilles
Tel.: 05 90 84 95 21
Fax: 05 90 84 60 87
Therapist: Fabiana de Oliveira
E-mail: allencaraibes@
wanadoo.fr

ALLEN CARR DENMARK

Website: www.easywaydk.dk

COPENHAGEN
Asger Rygsgade 16, 1th
1727 Copenhagen V
Tel.: 45 3331 0476
Mobile: 5190 3536
Therapist: Mette Fonss
E-mail: mettef@image.dk

ALLEN CARR ECUADOR

QUITO
Gaspar de Villarroel
E9–59y Av. Shyris
Quito
Tel. & Fax: 00593 2 2820 920
Therapist: Ingrid Wittich
E-mail: toisan@pi.pro.ec

ALLEN CARR FRANCE

Website: www.allencarr.fr

MARSEILLE
70 Rue St Ferreol
13006 Marseille
Freephone: 0800 15 57 40
Tel.: 04 91 33 54 55

Fax: 04 91 33 32 77
Therapist: Erick Serre
E-mail: info@allencarr.fr

PARIS
125 Boulevard Montparnasse
75006 Paris
Freephone: 0800 15 57 40
Tel.: 04 91 33 54 55
Therapist: Erick Serre

LANGUEDOC
1051 Rue de Las Sorbes
34070 Montpellier
Tel.: 0467 412960
Therapist: Dominique Hertogh

ROUSSILLON
1 Rue Pierre Curie
66000 Perpignan
Tel.: 04 68 34 40 68
Therapist: Eugene Salas
E-mail: eugenesalas@
    minitel.net

TOULOUSE
54 Avenue Crampel
31400 Toulouse
Tel.: 0800 15 57 40

ALLEN CARR
GERMANY

Website: www.allen-carr.de
E-mail: info@allen-carr.de

Free line telephone for
    Information:
0800 RAUCHEN (0800
    7282436)
Central Booking Line:
    01803 201717

Aussere Munchener Str. 34B
D-83026 Rosenheim
Tel.: 0049 8031 463067
Fax: 0049 8031 463068
Therapists: Erich Kellermann
    and team

ALLEN CARR
HOLLAND

Website: www.allencarr.nl
E-mail: amsterdam@
    allencarr.nl

AMSTERDAM
Pythagorasstraat 22
1098 GC Amsterdam
Tel.: 020 465 4665
Fax: 020 465 6682
Therapist: Eveline de Mooij
E-mail: amsterdam@
    allencarr.nl

UTRECHT
De Beaufortlaan 22B
3768 MJ Soestduinen
    (gem. Soest)
Tel.: 035 602 94 58
Therapist: Paula Rooduijn
E-mail: soest@allencarr.nl

ROTTERDAM
Mathenesserlaan 290
3021 HV Rotterdam
Tel.: 010 244 0709
Fax: 010 244 0710
Therapist: Kitty van't Hof
E-mail: rotterdam@
    allencarr.nl

NIJMEGEN
Dominicanenstraat 4

6521 KD Nijmegen
Tel.: 024 360 33 05
Therapist: Jacqueline van
  den Bosch
E-mail: nijmegen@
  allencarr.nl

ALLEN CARR ICELAND

REYKJAVIK
Ljosheimar 4
104 Reykjavik
Tel.: 354 553 9590
Fax: 354 588 7060
Therapists: Petur Einarsson &
  Valgeir Skagfjord
E-mail: easyway@simnet.is

ALLEN CARR ITALY

Website:
  www.easywayitalia.com

MILAN
Studio Pavanello
Piazza Argentina 4
20124 Milan
Mobile: 0348 354 7774 or
  0322 980 350
Therapist: Francesca Cesati
E-mail: fcesati@
  cableinet.co.uk
info@easywayitalia.com

ALLEN CARR NEW ZEALAND

AUCKLAND
472 Blockhouse Bay Road
Auckland 1007

Tel.: 09 626 5390
Mobile: 027 4177077
Therapist: Vickie Macrae
E-mail: macrazies@xtra.co.nz

ALLEN CARR PORTUGAL

OPORTO
Rua Fernandes Tomas
424–2° Sala 5
4000–210 Porto
Tel.: 351 225 102840
Fax: 351 229 407234
Therapist: Fatima Helder
  (weight clinic only)
E-mail: easyweigh@
  mail.telepac.pt
www.fatimahelder.com

Rua dos Castanheiros 97
4455–089 Lavra–Matosinhos
Tel.: 229 958698
Fax: 229 955507
Therapist: Ria Monteiro
E-mail: slofmont@
  mail.telepac.pt

ALLEN CARR SOUTH AFRICA

CAPETOWN
PO Box 5269
Helderberg
Somerset West 7135
Tel.: 083 8 600 5555
Fax: 083 8 600 5555
Therapist: Dr Charles Nel
E-mail: easyway@
  allencarr.co.za

ALLEN CARR SOUTH AMERICA

COLOMBIA
Cra. 9 No. 77–19
Bogota
Tel.: 571 313 3030 and
    571 211 7662
Therapists: Felipe Calderon,
    Jose Manuel Duran
E-mail: positron@cc-net.net

ALLEN CARR SPAIN

MADRID AND BARCELONA
Tel.: 902 10 28 10
Fax: 942 83 25 84
Therapists: Geoffrey Molloy,
    Rhea Sivi

E-mail: easyway@
    comodejardefumar.com

ALLEN CARR SWITZERLAND

Free line telephone for
    Information and Booking:
0800 RAUCHEN (0800
    7282426)
Schontalstrasse 30
Ch-8486 Zürich–Rikon
Tel.: 00 41 52 383 3773
Fax: 00 41 52 383 3774
Therapist: Cyrill Argast and
    team
E-mail: info@allen-carr.ch
Website: www.allen-carr.ch

ALLEN CARR'S EASY WAY TO STOP SMOKING

'If you follow my instructions, you will be happy to be a non-smoker for the rest of your life'
Allen Carr

Allen Carr's method is unique. Follow his guidelines to help you remove the psychological need to smoke – without scare tactics, weight gain or fear of deprivation. Learn how great it feels to be a non-smoker with help from an expert.

'One by one Allen Carr demolishes all the reasons why smokers cling to the habit' *Today*

'His skill is in removing the psychological dependence' *Sunday Times*

By the same author

THE ONLY WAY
TO STOP SMOKING
PERMANENTLY

Following the enormous success of his best-selling *Easy Way to Stop Smoking*, Allen Carr here exposes the traps of smoking and provides smokers with the motivation to break free for ever.

This book will help you:

• achieve the right frame of mind to quit

• ignore the myths of addiction, weight gain and willpower

• give up without dependence on rules or gimmicks

• enjoy the freedom and choices that non-smokers have in life

'A different approach ... a stunning success'
Sun

By the same author

HOW TO STOP YOUR CHILD SMOKING

In this book Allen Carr directs his common-sense methods at parents and children. It is, he asserts, by falling into the nicotine trap that the vast majority of smokers are introduced to the idea that they cannot enjoy life or cope with stress without taking chemical poisons. This straight-talking, sensible book is the key to achieving this aim and gives sound advice on:

• how to communicate freely and openly with your children

• recognizing that smoking is not a choice, but a trap

• resisting the pressure of friends, partners and advertising

• setting a good example

THE EASY WAY TO ENJOY FLYING

In this life-changing book Allen Carr turns his unique methods to fear of flying, a problem which affects thousands of people. *The Easy Way to Enjoy Flying* shows how fear of flying is nothing to be ashamed of, but is part of human nature – yet one which is ultimately based on misconceptions. Eliminating these misconceptions will remove the fear and enable you to enjoy flying to the full. This book:

• dispels our most common fears of flying

• explodes the media myths that surround flying

• removes the root of fear itself, unlike other relaxation methods, which concentrate on the symptoms of fear

refresh yourself at penguin.co.uk

Visit penguin.co.uk for exclusive information and interviews with
bestselling authors, fantastic give-aways and the
inside track on all our books, from the Penguin Classics
to the latest bestsellers.

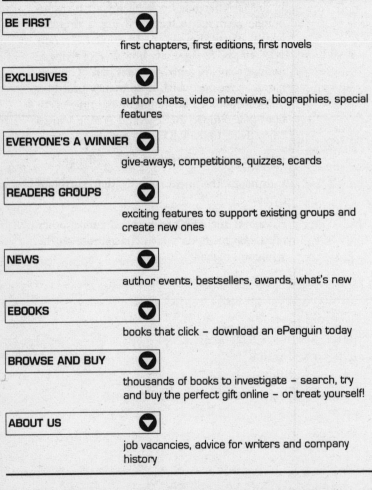

BE FIRST

first chapters, first editions, first novels

EXCLUSIVES

author chats, video interviews, biographies, special
features

EVERYONE'S A WINNER

give-aways, competitions, quizzes, ecards

READERS GROUPS

exciting features to support existing groups and
create new ones

NEWS

author events, bestsellers, awards, what's new

EBOOKS

books that click – download an ePenguin today

BROWSE AND BUY

thousands of books to investigate – search, try
and buy the perfect gift online – or treat yourself!

ABOUT US

job vacancies, advice for writers and company
history

Get Closer To Penguin . . . www.penguin.co.uk